THE HEALING
GOUT DIET
COOKBOOK
FOR BEGINNERS

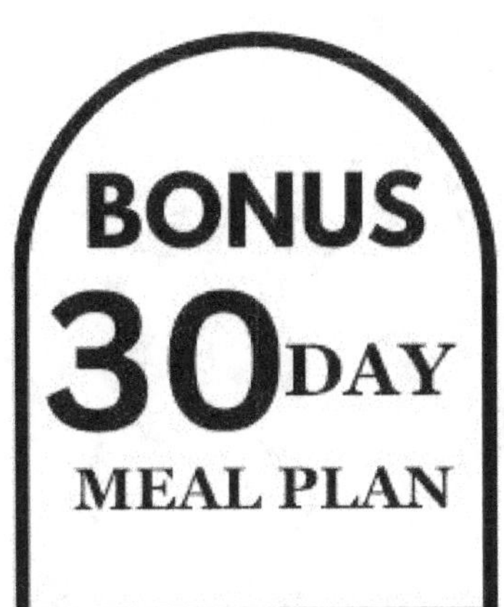

This Cookbook Belongs To:

Acknowledgments

I would like to express my heartfelt gratitude to all those who have contributed to the creation of this book on gout management.

First and foremost, I extend my deepest appreciation to the healthcare professionals who have dedicated their time, expertise, and compassion to caring for individuals with gout. Your unwavering commitment to improving the lives of patients is truly inspiring.

I am indebted to the individuals who generously shared their personal experiences and success stories of living with gout. Your courage, resilience, and willingness to share your journey have added depth and authenticity to this book.

I am thankful to my family, friends, and colleagues for their constant support, encouragement, and understanding throughout the process of writing this book. Your words of encouragement, constructive feedback, and patience have been invaluable.

I extend my gratitude to the authors, researchers, and organizations whose work has contributed to our understanding of gout and its management. Your dedication to advancing knowledge and raising awareness about gout is commendable.

I am grateful to the readers of this book for their interest in learning more about gout and their commitment to improving their health and well-being. It is my hope that this book will serve as a valuable resource and guide on their journey to managing gout effectively.

Thank you to everyone who has contributed to the creation of this book. Your support and collaboration have made this endeavor possible.

TABLE OF CONTENTS

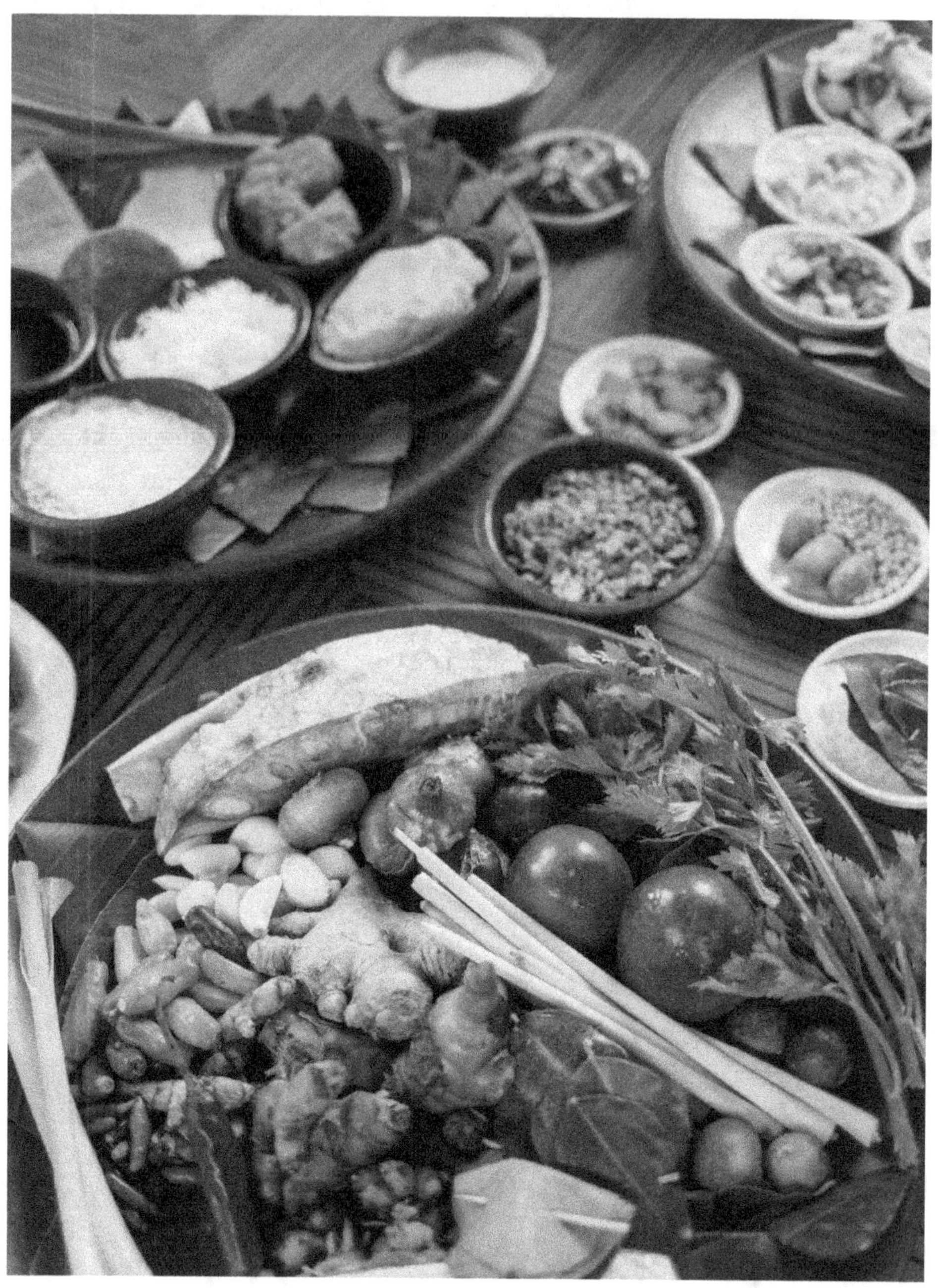

HERE'S YOUR 30 DAY MEAL PLAN BONUS

Day 1

- **Breakfast:** Oatmeal topped with strawberries and almonds
- **Lunch:** Spinach salad with grilled chicken, cherry tomatoes, and balsamic vinaigrette
- **Dinner:** Baked salmon with quinoa and steamed broccoli

Day 2

- **Breakfast:** Greek yogurt with sliced bananas and chia seeds
- **Lunch:** Lentil soup with whole wheat bread
- **Dinner:** Stir-fried tofu with mixed vegetables and brown rice

Day 3

- **Breakfast:** Whole grain toast with avocado and tomato slices
- **Lunch:** Chickpea salad with bell peppers, cucumbers, and lemon-tahini dressing
- **Dinner:** Grilled turkey burgers with sweet potato fries and green salad

Day 4

- **Breakfast:** Berry smoothie with spinach, almond milk, and flaxseeds
- **Lunch:** Quinoa salad with mixed greens, cherry tomatoes, and grilled shrimp
- **Dinner:** Eggplant and chickpea curry with brown rice

Day 5

- **Breakfast:** Scrambled eggs with sautéed spinach and whole grain toast

- **Lunch:** Black bean tacos with avocado, salsa, and lettuce wraps
- **Dinner:** Baked chicken breast with roasted cauliflower and quinoa pilaf

Day 6

- Breakfast: Overnight oats with diced apples and cinnamon
- Lunch: Tofu and vegetable stir-fry with brown rice
- Dinner: Grilled salmon with asparagus and wild rice

Day 7

- **Breakfast:** Greek yogurt parfait with mixed berries and granola
- **Lunch:** Lentil and vegetable soup with whole wheat crackers
- **Dinner:** Turkey meatballs with zucchini noodles and marinara sauce

Day 8

- **Breakfast:** Whole grain pancakes topped with sliced bananas and almond butter
- **Lunch:** Spinach salad with grilled chicken, strawberries, and balsamic vinaigrette
- **Dinner:** Baked cod with quinoa salad and steamed green beans

Day 9

- **Breakfast:** Smoothie bowl with spinach, pineapple, and coconut flakes
- **Lunch:** Quinoa and black bean salad with avocado, corn, and lime dressing
- **Dinner:** Stir-fried tofu with broccoli and bell peppers served over brown rice

Day 10

- **Breakfast:** Whole grain toast with mashed avocado and cherry tomatoes
- **Lunch:** Chickpea and vegetable curry with brown rice
- **Dinner:** Grilled turkey burgers with sweet potato fries and side salad

Day 11

- **Breakfast:** Greek yogurt with mixed berries and chia seeds
- **Lunch:** Lentil soup with whole wheat bread
- **Dinner:** Baked chicken breast with roasted Brussels sprouts and quinoa pilaf

Day 12

- **Breakfast**: Berry smoothie with spinach, almond milk, and flaxseeds
- **Lunch:** Quinoa salad with mixed greens, cherry tomatoes, and grilled shrimp
- **Dinner:** Eggplant and chickpea curry with brown rice

Day 13

- **Breakfast:** Scrambled eggs with sautéed spinach and whole grain toast
- **Lunch:** Black bean tacos with avocado, salsa, and lettuce wraps
- **Dinner:** Baked salmon with roasted cauliflower and wild rice

Day 14

- **Breakfast:** Overnight oats with diced apples and cinnamon
- **Lunch:** Tofu and vegetable stir-fry with brown rice
- **Dinner:** Turkey meatballs with zucchini noodles and marinara sauce

Day 15

- **Breakfast:** Greek yogurt parfait with mixed berries and granola
- **Lunch:** Lentil and vegetable soup with whole wheat crackers
- **Dinner:** Grilled cod with quinoa salad and steamed green beans

Day 16

- **Breakfast:** Whole grain pancakes topped with sliced bananas and almond butter
- **Lunch:** Spinach salad with grilled chicken, strawberries, and balsamic vinaigrette
- **Dinner:** Baked cod with quinoa salad and steamed green beans

Day 17

- **Breakfast:** Smoothie bowl with spinach, pineapple, and coconut flakes
- **Lunch:** Quinoa and black bean salad with avocado, corn, and lime dressing
- **Dinner:** Stir-fried tofu with broccoli and bell peppers served over brown rice

Day 18

- **Breakfast:** Whole grain toast with mashed avocado and cherry tomatoes
- **Lunch:** Chickpea and vegetable curry with brown rice
- **Dinner:** Grilled turkey burgers with sweet potato fries and side salad

Day 19:

- **Breakfast:** Greek yogurt with mixed berries and chia seeds
- **Lunch:** Lentil soup with whole wheat bread

- **Dinner:** Baked chicken breast with roasted Brussels sprouts and quinoa pilaf

Day 20

- **Breakfast:** Berry smoothie with spinach, almond milk, and flaxseeds
- **Lunch:** Quinoa salad with mixed greens, cherry tomatoes, and grilled shrimp
- **Dinner:** Eggplant and chickpea curry with brown rice

Day 21

- **Breakfast:** Scrambled eggs with sautéed spinach and whole grain toast
- **Lunch:** Black bean tacos with avocado, salsa, and lettuce wraps
- **Dinner:** Baked salmon with roasted cauliflower and wild rice

Day 22

- **Breakfast:** Overnight oats with diced apples and cinnamon
- **Lunch:** Tofu and vegetable stir-fry with brown rice
- **Dinner:** Turkey meatballs with zucchini noodles and marinara sauce

Day 23

- **Breakfast:** Greek yogurt parfait with mixed berries and granola
- **Lunch:** Lentil and vegetable soup with whole wheat crackers
- **Dinner:** Grilled cod with quinoa salad and steamed green beans

Day 24

- **Breakfast:** Whole grain pancakes topped with sliced bananas and almond butter

- **Lunch:** Spinach salad with grilled chicken, strawberries, and balsamic vinaigrette
- **Dinner:** Baked cod with quinoa salad and steamed green beans

Day 25

- **Breakfast:** Smoothie bowl with spinach, pineapple, and coconut flakes
- **Lunch:** Quinoa and black bean salad with avocado, corn, and lime dressing
- **Dinner:** Stir-fried tofu with broccoli and bell peppers served over brown rice

Day 26

- **Breakfast:** Whole grain toast with mashed avocado and cherry tomatoes
- **Lunch:** Chickpea and vegetable curry with brown rice
- **Dinner:** Grilled turkey burgers with sweet potato fries and side salad

Day 27

- **Breakfast:** Greek yogurt with mixed berries and chia seeds
- **Lunch:** Lentil soup with whole wheat bread
- **Dinner:** Baked chicken breast with roasted Brussels sprouts and quinoa pilaf

Day 28

- **Breakfast:** Berry smoothie with spinach, almond milk, and flaxseeds
- **Lunch:** Quinoa salad with mixed greens, cherry tomatoes, and grilled shrimp

- **Dinner:** Eggplant and chickpea curry with brown rice

Day 29
- **Breakfast:** Scrambled eggs with sautéed spinach and whole grain toast
- **Lunch:** Black bean tacos with avocado, salsa, and lettuce wraps
- **Dinner:** Baked salmon with roasted cauliflower and wild rice

Day 30
- **Breakfast:** Overnight oats with diced apples and cinnamon
- **Lunch:** Tofu and vegetable stir-fry with brown rice
- **Dinner:** Turkey meatballs with zucchini noodles and marinara sauce

Continue this meal plan pattern for as many days you want to, ensuring variety in your meals and incorporating a range of fruits, vegetables, whole grains, lean proteins, and healthy fats. Remember to drink plenty of water throughout the day to stay hydrated and support kidney function. Additionally, listen to your body's hunger and fullness cues, and adjust portion sizes as needed.

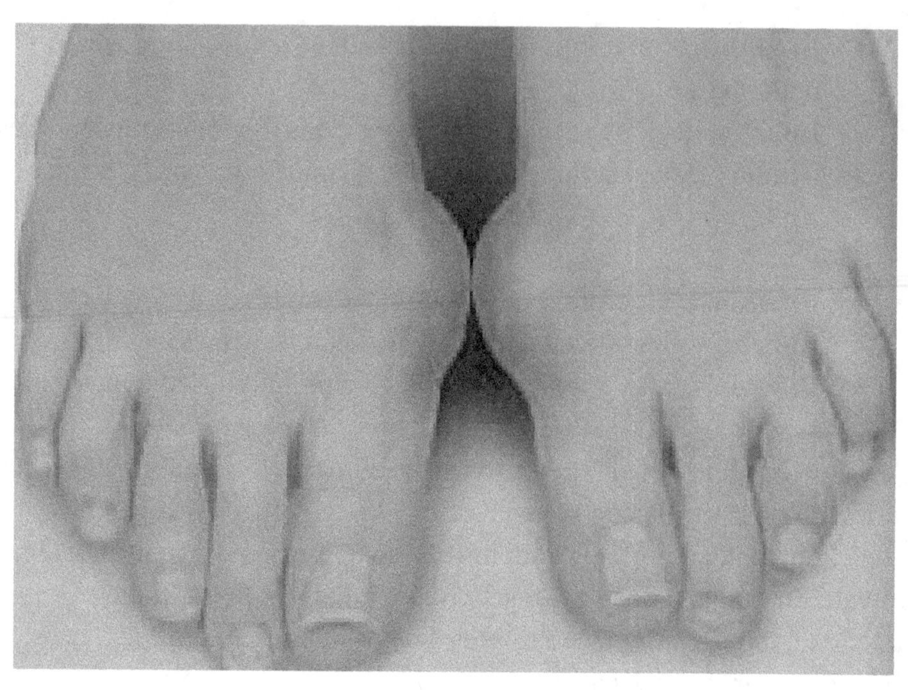

INTRODUCTION

About This Book

Welcome to The Healing Gout Diet Cookbook for beginners! Whether you're newly diagnosed with gout or seeking effective ways to manage your condition, this book is designed to provide you with practical guidance and support on navigating the gout diet and lifestyle.

Gout is a form of arthritis that can cause intense pain and discomfort, often affecting the joints, particularly in the feet. While there is no cure for gout, managing the condition through lifestyle changes, including diet modifications, can help reduce the frequency and severity of flare-ups and improve overall quality of life.

In this book, you'll find a comprehensive overview of gout, including its causes, symptoms, and complications, as well as a detailed exploration of the role of diet in gout management. You'll learn about the foods that can help alleviate symptoms and those that can exacerbate them, along with practical tips for creating delicious and satisfying meals that support your gout-friendly lifestyle.

Beyond diet, we'll also delve into other important aspects of gout management, such as exercise, weight management, stress reduction, and the use of supplements and natural remedies. Additionally, you'll find guidance on recognizing and managing gout flares, as well as answers to common questions and concerns about the condition.

Throughout this book, our goal is to empower you with the knowledge and tools you need to take control of your gout and live your life to the fullest. Whether you're just starting your journey or looking for new strategies to enhance your gout management plan, we hope you'll find this book to be a valuable resource.

Thank you for joining us on this journey toward better health and well-being. Let's embark on this path together, one step at a time.

What is Gout?

Gout is a type of arthritis characterized by sudden and severe attacks of pain, swelling, redness, and tenderness in the joints, most commonly the big toe. It occurs when urate crystals accumulate in the joints, leading to inflammation and intense discomfort.

Urate crystals form when there is an excess of uric acid in the bloodstream, a condition known as hyperuricemia. Uric acid is a waste product that is normally dissolved in the blood and excreted from the body through urine. However, in some individuals, the body produces too much uric acid or has difficulty eliminating it, leading to elevated levels in the blood and the formation of crystals in the joints.

Gout attacks often occur suddenly and can be triggered by factors such as:

Diet: Consuming foods high in purines, such as red meat, shellfish, and certain types of alcohol, can increase uric acid levels and trigger gout attacks.

Lifestyle factors: Obesity, dehydration, and excessive alcohol consumption can also contribute to the development of gout.

Genetics: Family history and genetic predisposition can play a role in the development of gout.

Medical conditions: Certain medical conditions, such as kidney disease, diabetes, and high blood pressure, can increase the risk of gout.

While gout primarily affects the joints, it can also cause other health complications if left untreated, including kidney stones, kidney damage, and joint damage.

Managing gout typically involves a combination of lifestyle changes, such as following a gout-friendly diet, maintaining a healthy weight, staying hydrated, and avoiding triggers, as well as medications to reduce inflammation and lower uric acid levels in the blood.

By understanding the underlying causes and triggers of gout and taking proactive steps to manage the condition, individuals can reduce the frequency and severity of gout attacks and improve their overall quality of life.

The Importance of Diet in Managing Gout

Diet plays a crucial role in the management of gout, as certain foods can either help alleviate symptoms or exacerbate them by influencing uric acid levels in the body. Understanding which foods to include in a gout-friendly diet and which to avoid can help individuals with gout reduce the frequency and severity of flare-ups and improve overall health.

Foods to Include

Low-Purine Foods: Purines are substances found in certain foods that can break down into uric acid in the body. Choosing foods that are low in purines can help reduce uric acid levels and minimize the risk of gout attacks. Examples of low-purine foods include fruits, vegetables, whole grains, legumes, nuts, and seeds.

High-Fiber Foods: Fiber-rich foods, such as fruits, vegetables, whole grains, and legumes, can help regulate uric acid levels by promoting healthy digestion and elimination. They also provide essential nutrients and support overall health.

Healthy Fats: Incorporating sources of healthy fats, such as olive oil, avocados, nuts, and fatty fish like salmon, can help reduce inflammation and support heart health. Omega-3 fatty acids, in particular, have been shown to have anti-inflammatory properties and may help reduce the risk of gout flares.

Low-Fat Dairy: Low-fat dairy products, such as milk, yogurt, and cheese, may help lower uric acid levels and reduce the risk of gout attacks. Calcium and vitamin D, which are found in dairy products, may also have protective effects against gout.

Foods to Avoid or Limit

High-Purine Foods: Foods that are high in purines can increase uric acid levels in the body and trigger gout attacks. Examples of high-purine foods include red meat, organ meats (such as liver and kidney), shellfish, and certain types of alcohol (especially beer and liquor).

Processed Foods and Sugary Beverages: Processed foods, sugary beverages, and foods high in refined carbohydrates can contribute to weight gain and increase the risk of gout flares. Limiting intake of these foods can help manage gout symptoms and support overall health.

Alcohol: Alcohol consumption, especially beer and liquor, can increase uric acid levels and trigger gout attacks. Reducing or eliminating alcohol intake, particularly during gout flares, can help prevent recurrence of symptoms.

Sugary Foods and Beverages: High intake of sugary foods and beverages, such as soda, candy, and desserts, has been associated with an increased risk of gout. Limiting consumption of these items can help control uric acid levels and reduce the frequency of gout attacks.

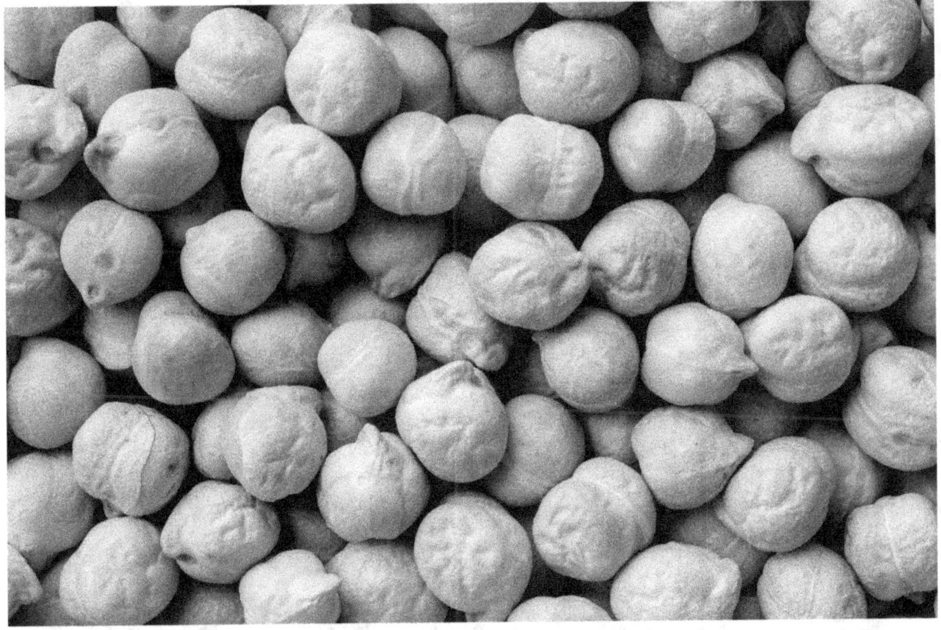

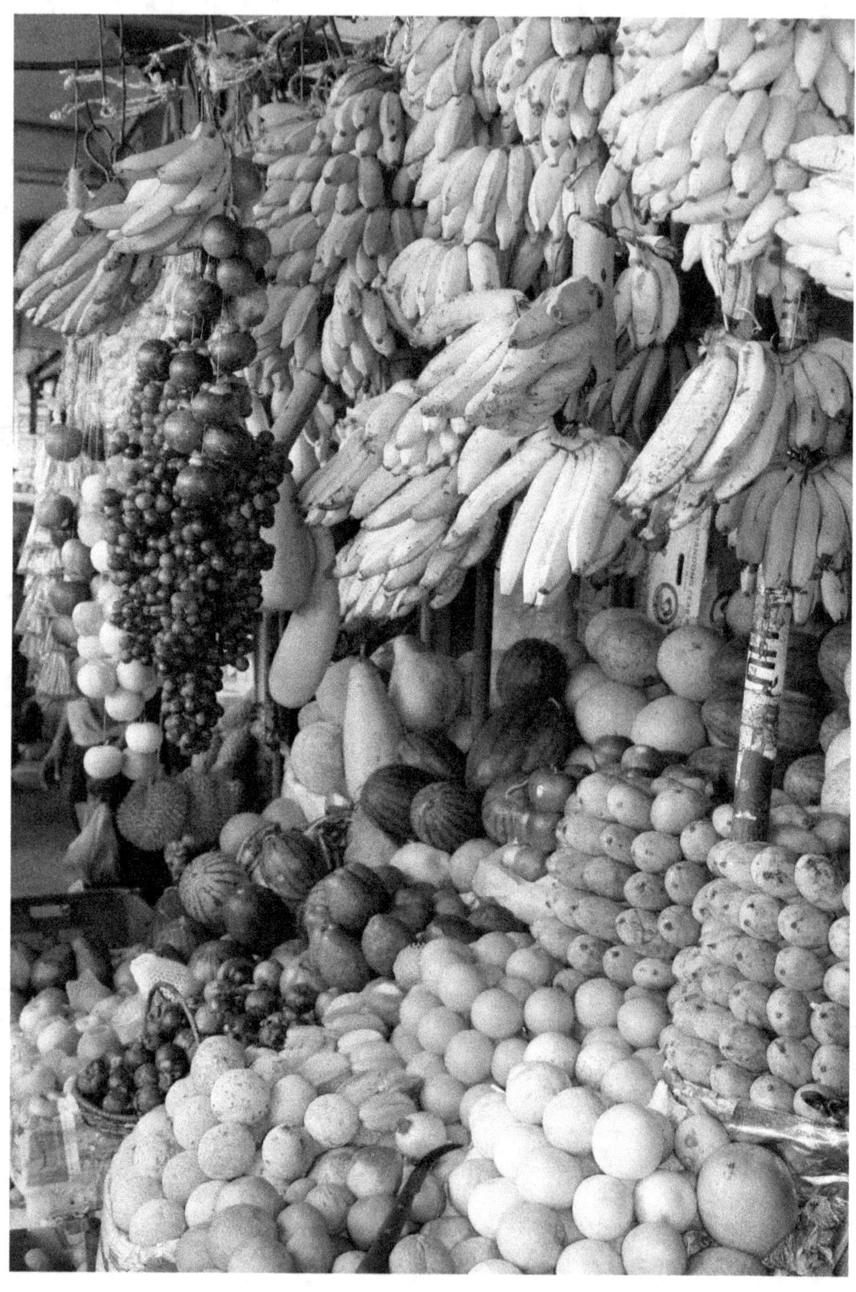

CHAPTER ONE

Understanding Gout

What is Gout?

Gout is a type of inflammatory arthritis characterized by sudden and severe attacks of pain, swelling, redness, and tenderness in the joints, most commonly in the big toe. It occurs when urate crystals accumulate in the joints, leading to inflammation and intense discomfort.

Urate crystals form when there is an excess of uric acid in the bloodstream, a condition known as hyperuricemia. Uric acid is a waste product that is normally dissolved in the blood and excreted from the body through urine. However, in some individuals, the body produces too much uric acid or has difficulty eliminating it, leading to elevated levels in the blood and the formation of crystals in the joints.

Gout attacks often occur suddenly and can be triggered by factors such as diet, lifestyle, genetics, and underlying medical conditions. Foods high in purines, such as red meat, shellfish, and certain types of alcohol, can increase uric acid levels and trigger gout attacks. Other risk factors for gout include obesity, dehydration, excessive alcohol consumption, family history of gout, and certain medical conditions like kidney disease and high blood pressure.

While gout primarily affects the joints, it can also cause other health complications if left untreated, including kidney stones, kidney damage, and joint damage.

Managing gout typically involves a combination of lifestyle changes, such as following a gout-friendly diet, maintaining a healthy weight, staying hydrated, and avoiding triggers, as well as medications to reduce inflammation and lower uric acid levels in the blood.

By understanding the underlying causes and triggers of gout and taking proactive steps to manage the condition, individuals can reduce the frequency and severity of gout attacks and improve their overall quality of life.

Causes and Risk Factors of Gout

Gout is caused by the accumulation of urate crystals in the joints, resulting in inflammation and pain. Urate crystals form when there is an excess of uric acid in the bloodstream, a condition known as hyperuricemia. Several factors can contribute to the development of hyperuricemia and gout, including:

1. Diet: Consuming foods high in purines can increase uric acid levels in the blood and contribute to the formation of urate crystals. Foods high in purines include red meat, organ meats (such as liver and kidney), shellfish, and certain types of alcohol, particularly beer and liquor.

2. Lifestyle Factors: Certain lifestyle factors can increase the risk of developing gout. These include:

Obesity: Excess body weight can lead to higher uric acid levels and increase the risk of gout.

Dehydration: Inadequate hydration can lead to higher concentrations of uric acid in the blood and increase the risk of gout attacks.

Alcohol consumption: Alcohol, especially beer and liquor, can increase uric acid levels and trigger gout attacks.

3. Genetics: Family history and genetic predisposition can play a role in the development of gout. Some people inherit genetic variations that affect how their bodies produce or eliminate uric acid, increasing their risk of hyperuricemia and gout.

4. Medical Conditions: Certain medical conditions can increase the risk of developing gout. These include:

Kidney disease: Impaired kidney function can lead to reduced uric acid excretion and increase the risk of hyperuricemia and gout.

High blood pressure: Hypertension is associated with an increased risk of gout, possibly due to its effects on kidney function.

Diabetes: Insulin resistance and obesity associated with type 2 diabetes can contribute to higher uric acid levels and increase the risk of gout.

5. Medications: Some medications can increase uric acid levels in the blood and contribute to the development of gout. These include diuretics (water pills) used to treat hypertension and certain immune-suppressing drugs.

6. Gender and Age: Gout is more common in men than women, particularly in middle-aged and older adults. However, women's risk of developing gout increases after menopause, when estrogen levels decrease.

By understanding the causes and risk factors of gout, individuals can take proactive steps to reduce their risk and manage the condition effectively through lifestyle changes, dietary modifications, and medical treatment when necessary.

Symptoms of Gout

Gout is characterized by sudden and intense attacks of pain, swelling, redness, warmth, and tenderness in the joints, most commonly in the big toe. These symptoms typically come on rapidly, often overnight, and can be extremely debilitating. The signs and symptoms of gout may include:

Joint Pain: The hallmark symptom of gout is severe joint pain, usually in the big toe. However, gout can also affect other joints, such as the ankles, knees, elbows, wrists, and fingers. The pain is often described as excruciating and may be throbbing, stabbing, or burning in nature.

Swelling: The affected joint may become swollen and inflamed, making it appear larger than usual. The swelling may be accompanied by redness and warmth in the area.

Redness: The skin over the affected joint may appear red or purplish in color due to inflammation and increased blood flow to the area.

Tenderness: The joint may be extremely tender to the touch, and even the slightest pressure or movement can cause intense pain.

Limited Range of Motion: During a gout attack, movement of the affected joint may be restricted due to pain and swelling.

Fever: In some cases, gout attacks may be accompanied by a low-grade fever.

Gout attacks typically last for a few days to a week or longer, with symptoms gradually subsiding over time. However, without proper treatment and management, gout attacks may recur frequently and become more severe over time, leading to chronic gout and joint damage.

It's important to note that not everyone with hyperuricemia (elevated uric acid levels) will experience gout symptoms. Some individuals may have high uric acid levels for years without developing gout, while others may experience gout attacks despite having normal or only slightly elevated uric acid levels.

If you experience symptoms of gout, it's essential to seek medical attention for an accurate diagnosis and appropriate treatment. Untreated gout can lead to complications such as kidney stones, joint damage, and chronic arthritis.

Complications of Untreated Gout

Recurrent Gout Attacks: Without proper management, gout attacks can recur frequently and become more severe over time. Each subsequent attack may last longer and affect multiple joints, leading to increased pain and disability.

Joint Damage: Chronic inflammation from untreated gout can damage the affected joints over time, leading to joint deformities, decreased mobility, and loss of function. Severe cases of gout may result in permanent joint damage and disability.

Tophi Formation: Tophi are deposits of urate crystals that accumulate in the joints, tendons, and surrounding tissues over time. These chalky nodules can cause swelling, deformity, and chronic pain, and may eventually erode the affected tissues if left untreated.

Kidney Stones: High levels of uric acid in the blood can lead to the formation of urate crystals in the kidneys, resulting in the development of kidney stones. These small, hard deposits can cause intense pain and may require medical intervention to manage.

Kidney Damage: Chronic hyperuricemia and recurrent gout attacks can contribute to kidney damage over time. Urate crystals can accumulate in the kidneys, leading to inflammation, scarring, and impaired kidney function. Untreated gout is associated with an increased risk of chronic kidney disease and kidney failure.

Cardiovascular Disease: There is growing evidence to suggest that gout may be associated with an increased risk of cardiovascular disease, including heart attacks, strokes, and high blood pressure. Chronic inflammation from untreated gout may contribute to the development and progression of cardiovascular complications.

Joint Infections: In severe cases of untreated gout, the inflamed and damaged joints may become susceptible to bacterial infections. Joint infections can cause additional pain, swelling, and complications, and may require antibiotics or surgical intervention to treat.

Chronic Pain and Disability: Persistent gout symptoms and complications can have a significant impact on quality of life, leading to chronic pain, disability, and reduced mobility. Individuals with untreated gout may experience limitations in daily activities and diminished overall well-being.

It's important to seek medical attention and treatment for gout as soon as symptoms develop to prevent complications and improve long-term outcomes. With proper management, including lifestyle changes, medication, and regular monitoring, most people with gout can effectively control their symptoms and reduce the risk of complications.

CHAPTER TWO

The Gout Diet Explained

The Role of Diet in Gout Management

Diet plays a significant role in managing gout by helping to control uric acid levels in the bloodstream. By making dietary changes and adopting healthy eating habits, individuals with gout can reduce the frequency and severity of gout attacks and improve overall health. Here are some key dietary considerations for managing gout:

1. Avoid High-Purine Foods

Purines are compounds found in certain foods that can increase uric acid levels in the blood, leading to gout attacks. Foods high in purines include red meat, organ meats (such as liver and kidneys), shellfish, and certain types of alcohol, particularly beer and liquor. Limiting or avoiding these foods can help reduce the risk of gout attacks.

2. Choose Low-Purine Foods

Opt for foods that are low in purines, such as fruits, vegetables, whole grains, legumes, nuts, and seeds. These foods are less likely to contribute to elevated uric acid levels and can be included as part of a gout-friendly diet.

3. Stay Hydrated

Drinking plenty of water and staying hydrated is essential for managing gout. Adequate hydration helps to dilute uric acid in the blood and promote its excretion through urine. Aim to drink at least 8-10 cups of water per day, and limit intake of sugary beverages and alcohol, which can contribute to dehydration.

4. Maintain a Healthy Weight

Obesity and excess body weight are risk factors for gout and can exacerbate symptoms. Losing weight through a combination of diet and exercise can help reduce uric acid levels and decrease the frequency of gout attacks. Focus on adopting a balanced diet rich in fruits, vegetables, lean proteins, and whole grains, and incorporate regular physical activity into your routine.

5. Limit Alcohol Intake

Alcohol consumption, especially beer and liquor, can increase uric acid levels in the blood and trigger gout attacks. If you drink alcohol, do so in moderation and avoid binge drinking. Limiting alcohol intake can help reduce the risk of gout flares and improve overall gout management.

6. Monitor Portion Sizes

Pay attention to portion sizes and avoid overeating, especially high-purine foods. Eating large portions of high-purine foods can increase uric acid levels in the blood and contribute to gout attacks. Aim for balanced, portion-controlled meals and snacks to maintain a healthy weight and support gout management.

7. Consider Dietary Supplements

Some dietary supplements, such as vitamin C and cherry extract, have been suggested to have potential benefits for gout management. Talk to your healthcare provider before taking any supplements to ensure they are safe and appropriate for you.

By making smart dietary choices and adopting a gout-friendly eating plan, individuals with gout can effectively manage their symptoms and reduce the risk of gout attacks. It's essential to work with a healthcare provider or registered dietitian to develop a personalized diet plan that meets your individual needs and goals.

Understanding Purines and Uric Acid

1. What are Purines?

Purines are natural compounds found in many foods and beverages. They are essential components of DNA, RNA, and ATP (adenosine triphosphate), which play vital roles in cellular function and energy metabolism.

2. Uric Acid Production

When purines are broken down in the body, they produce a waste product called uric acid. Uric acid is normally dissolved in the blood and excreted from the body through urine. However, in some individuals, uric acid levels can become elevated, leading to hyperuricemia.

3. Hyperuricemia

Hyperuricemia is a condition characterized by high levels of uric acid in the bloodstream. It can occur due to various factors, including genetics, dietary habits, obesity, certain medical conditions, and medications. When uric acid levels exceed the body's ability to excrete it, urate crystals can form in the joints and surrounding tissues, leading to inflammation and gout attacks.

4. Role of Diet

Diet plays a significant role in determining uric acid levels in the body. Foods high in purines, such as red meat, organ meats (like liver and kidneys), shellfish, and certain types of alcohol (particularly beer and liquor), can contribute to elevated uric acid levels and increase the risk of gout attacks. Conversely, consuming foods low in purines, such as fruits, vegetables, whole grains, legumes, nuts, and seeds, can help reduce uric acid levels and support gout management.

5. Importance of Hydration

Staying hydrated is essential for managing uric acid levels in the body. Adequate hydration helps to dilute uric acid in the blood and promote its excretion through urine. Drinking plenty of water and limiting intake of sugary beverages and alcohol can help prevent dehydration and reduce the risk of gout attacks.

6. Monitoring Uric Acid Levels

Individuals with gout or hyperuricemia may undergo periodic blood tests to monitor uric acid levels. These tests can help healthcare providers assess disease activity, adjust treatment plans, and identify factors that may be contributing to elevated uric acid levels, such as diet, medications, or underlying medical conditions.

7. Treatment and Management

Managing gout typically involves a combination of lifestyle changes, dietary modifications, medication, and regular monitoring. By adopting a gout-friendly diet that limits purine-rich foods, staying hydrated, maintaining a healthy weight, and following prescribed treatment regimens, individuals with gout can effectively manage their symptoms and reduce the frequency of gout attacks.

Understanding the relationship between purines, uric acid, and gout is essential for effectively managing the condition and improving overall quality of life. By making smart dietary choices and working closely with healthcare providers, individuals with gout can take control of their health and reduce the impact of this chronic condition.

Foods to Include in a Gout Diet

1. Fruits

- Berries (e.g., strawberries, blueberries, raspberries)
- Cherries

- Apples
- Pears
- Pineapple
- Watermelon
- Citrus fruits (e.g., oranges, grapefruits)

2. Vegetables

- Leafy greens (e.g., spinach, kale, lettuce)
- Bell peppers
- Cucumbers
- Broccoli
- Cauliflower
- Carrots
- Tomatoes (in moderation)

3. Whole Grains

- Oats
- Quinoa
- Brown rice
- Barley
- Whole wheat products (e.g., bread, pasta)

4. Legumes

- Lentils
- Chickpeas
- Black beans
- Kidney beans
- Peas

5. Nuts and Seeds

- Almonds
- Walnuts
- Flaxseeds
- Chia seeds

6. Dairy
- Low-fat or fat-free dairy products (e.g., milk, yogurt, cheese)

7. Lean Proteins
- Poultry (e.g., chicken, turkey)
- Fish (especially fatty fish like salmon and trout)
- Tofu
- Eggs (in moderation)

8. Beverages
- Water
- Herbal teas
- Coffee (in moderation)

9. Cooking Oils
- Olive oil
- Avocado oil

10. Spices and Herbs
- Turmeric
- Ginger
- Garlic
- Cilantro
- Basil
- Parsley

11. Dairy Alternatives
- Plant-based milk alternatives (e.g., almond milk, soy milk)

12. Snacks
- Popcorn (air-popped)
- Fresh fruit
- Nuts and seeds (in moderation)

Note: Moderation is Key

While these foods are generally considered safe for a gout diet, it's essential to practice moderation and be mindful of portion sizes. Additionally, individual responses to specific foods may vary, so it's important to pay attention to your body and make adjustments based on how certain foods affect you.

It's also advisable to consult with a healthcare professional or a registered dietitian to create a personalized gout diet plan that takes into account your specific health needs, preferences, and any potential interactions with medications.

Remember, a gout-friendly diet is just one aspect of managing gout. Lifestyle factors, hydration, and medications prescribed by your healthcare provider also play crucial roles in preventing gout flares and maintaining overall health.

Always consult with your healthcare provider or a registered dietitian before making significant changes to your diet, especially if you have underlying health conditions or are taking medications.

Foods to Avoid or Limit for Gout Management

Gout is a type of arthritis caused by the buildup of urate crystals in the joints, resulting in inflammation and pain. While genetics and other factors play a role in the development of gout, dietary choices can significantly impact uric acid levels in the body. Certain foods are high in purines, compounds that break down into uric acid, and can contribute to gout attacks. To help manage gout symptoms and reduce the frequency of flare-ups, it's important to avoid or limit the following foods:

1. High-Purine Meats

Red meat, such as beef, lamb, and pork, is high in purines and should be limited in the diet of individuals with gout. Organ meats, such as liver, kidney, and sweetbreads, are particularly high in purines and should be avoided.

2. Shellfish

Shellfish, including shrimp, crab, lobster, and scallops, are rich in purines and can increase uric acid levels in the blood. Individuals with gout should limit their intake of shellfish to reduce the risk of gout attacks.

3. Certain Types of Alcohol

Beer and liquor, especially beer, are high in purines and can trigger gout attacks in susceptible individuals. Wine is generally considered to have a lower purine content and may be a better choice for those with gout, but moderation is still advised.

4. Sugary Beverages

Sugary beverages, such as soda, fruit juice, and sweetened teas, can contribute to weight gain and increase the risk of gout attacks. These beverages provide empty calories and can lead to dehydration, both of which can exacerbate gout symptoms.

5. Processed Foods and Sweets

Processed foods, including packaged snacks, fast food, and desserts, often contain high levels of refined carbohydrates, sugars, and unhealthy fats, which can contribute to inflammation and weight gain. Limiting intake of these foods can help manage gout symptoms and improve overall health.

6. High-Fructose Foods

Foods and beverages high in fructose, such as sugary snacks, desserts, and sweetened drinks, can increase uric acid levels in the blood and contribute to gout attacks. Fructose is metabolized into purines in the body, making it important to limit consumption for individuals with gout.

7. Certain Vegetables

While most vegetables are low in purines and can be included in a gout-friendly diet, some vegetables are higher in purines and should be consumed in moderation. These include spinach, asparagus, mushrooms, and cauliflower. However, these vegetables provide valuable nutrients and can still be enjoyed as part of a balanced diet.

8. High-Fat Dairy Products

High-fat dairy products, such as whole milk, cheese, and ice cream, can contribute to weight gain and increase the risk of gout attacks. Opt for low-fat or fat-free dairy options to reduce saturated fat intake and support gout management.

9. Excessive Salt

Consuming excessive salt can contribute to fluid retention and increase blood pressure, both of which can exacerbate gout symptoms. Limiting intake of high-sodium foods, such as processed meats, canned soups, and salty snacks, can help reduce inflammation and support overall health.

10. Fried Foods

Fried foods, such as french fries, fried chicken, and potato chips, are high in unhealthy fats and calories and can contribute to weight gain and inflammation. Limiting intake of fried foods can help manage gout symptoms and improve overall health.

By avoiding or limiting these high-purine and inflammatory foods and focusing on a diet rich in fruits, vegetables, whole grains, lean proteins, and low-fat dairy, individuals with gout can help reduce the frequency and severity of gout attacks and improve their overall quality of life.

FOOD CATEGORIES

Breakfast Recipes

Berry Oatmeal Bowl

Ingredients:

1 cup rolled oats.

2 cups of water or low-fat milk.

1 cup mixed berries (blueberries, strawberries, and raspberries).

1 tablespoon of chia seeds.

1 tablespoon honey or maple syrup.

A pinch of cinnamon.

Method of preparation:

1. Boil liquid: Bring a saucepan of water or milk to a boil.
2. Cook oats: Add the oats, decrease the heat to a simmer, and cook until soft (5 minutes).
3. Add Ingredients: Combine the mixed berries, chia seeds, and cinnamon.
4. Serve in a bowl, drizzled with honey or maple syrup.

Nutritional Value per Serving:

- Calories: 320.
- Protein: 9 grams.
- Carbohydrate: 60 grams
- Fat: 7g
- Fiber: 9 grams.

Serving Size: One bowl.

Time of preparation: Ten minutes.

Avocado toast with tomato.

Ingredients:

2 pieces of whole grain bread.

1 ripe avocado.

1 small, sliced tomato

Add salt and pepper to taste.

1 teaspoon of lemon juice.

fresh basil leaves (optional)

Method of preparation:

1. Toast the bread. Toast the bread pieces to the desired crispness.
2. Prepare the Avocado: Mash the avocado in a bowl with lemon juice, salt, and pepper.
3. Assemble by spreading mashed avocado on toasted bread and topping with tomato slices.
4. Garnish with fresh basil leaves, if preferred.

Nutritional Value per Serving:

- Calories: 350.
- Protein: 8 grams.
- Carbohydrate: 42g
- Fat: 18g
- Fiber: 10 grams.

Serving Size: One serving (2 slices).

Time of preparation: Ten minutes.

Spinach and Mushroom Omelette

Ingredients:

4 egg whites.

1 cup of fresh spinach leaves.

1/2 cup sliced mushrooms.

1/4 cup shredded low-fat cheese (such as mozzarella)

1 tablespoon of olive oil.

Add salt and pepper to taste.

Method of preparation:

1. Sauté vegetables. In a medium-sized pan, heat the olive oil. Sauté the mushrooms till golden, then add the spinach until wilted.
2. Whisk egg whites: In a mixing dish, combine egg whites with salt and pepper.
3. Cook an omelette: Cook until the egg whites are set, then sprinkle cheese on half of the omelette.
4. Fold: Fold the omelette in half and cook for an additional minute.

Nutritional Value per Serving:

- Calories: 180
- Protein: 20 grams
- Carbohydrate: 5 grams
- Fat: 9g
- Fiber: 2 grams.

Serving Size: One omelette

Time for preparation: 15 minutes.

Banana-Almond Smoothie

Ingredients:

One ripe banana.

1 cup of unsweetened almond milk.

1 tablespoon almond butter.

1 tablespoon of chia seeds.

One teaspoon honey (optional)

1/2 teaspoon of vanilla essence.

Ice cubes (Optional)

Method of preparation:

1. Blend: Blend all of the ingredients until smooth.
2. Adjust: If you like a thicker texture, add ice cubes.
3. Serve: Pour into a glass and enjoy.

Nutritional Value per Serving:

- Calories: 250.
- Protein: 5 grams.
- Carbs: 36g
- Fat: 11g
- Fiber: 6 grams.

Serving Size: One smoothie

Time of preparation: 5 minutes.

Chia Seed Pudding with Mango

Ingredients:

1/4 cup chia seeds.

1 cup almond or coconut milk.

1 tablespoon honey or maple syrup.

One ripe mango, sliced

1 teaspoon of vanilla essence.

Method of preparation:

1. Mix Chia Pudding: In a mixing dish, add chia seeds, milk, honey, and vanilla extract. Stir thoroughly.
2. Refrigerate: Cover and chill overnight or at least 4 hours until thickened.
3. Add mango: Before serving, top with the chopped mango.

Nutritional Value per Serving:
- Calories: 300.
- Protein: 6 grams.
- Carbs: 39g
- Fat: 15g
- Fiber: 11 grams.

Serving Size: One bowl.

Time of preparation: 10 minutes (plus chilling time).

These dishes are not only gout-friendly, but also quick and simple to make, making them ideal for hectic mornings! Please let me know if you want any further support or other recipes!

Lunch Recipes

Quinoa and Black Bean Salad Recipe

1 cup quinoa.

2 glasses of water.

1 can (15 oz) of black beans, drained and rinsed

1 cup cherry tomatoes, halved

One red bell pepper, chopped

1/4 cup red onion, finely chopped

1/4 cup of fresh cilantro, chopped

One avocado, diced

1/4 cup lime juice.

2 tablespoons of olive oil.

Add salt and pepper to taste.

Method of preparation:

1. Cook Quinoa: Rinse the quinoa under cool water. In a saucepan, mix the quinoa and water, then bring to a boil. Reduce the heat to low and cover. Cook for 15 minutes, or until the water is absorbed. Fluff with a fork and allow to cool.
2. Mix Salad: In a large mixing bowl, add cooked quinoa, black beans, cherry tomatoes, red bell pepper, red onion, and cilantro.
3. Dress Salad: In a small bowl, combine lime juice, olive oil, salt, and pepper. Pour over the salad and stir thoroughly.
4. Add avocados: Gently fold in the cubed avocado before serving.

Nutritional Value per Serving:
- Calories: 320.
- Protein: 9 grams.
- Carbohydrate: 42g
- Fat: 14g
- Fiber: 12 grams.

Serving Size: Four servings.
Time to Prepare: 20 minutes

Grilled Chicken and Avocado Wrap

Ingredients:
2 boneless and skinless chicken breasts.
2 tablespoons of olive oil.
1 teaspoon of paprika.
Add salt and pepper to taste.
Four whole wheat tortillas.
One avocado, sliced
1 cup mixed greens.
1/2 cup cherry tomatoes (halved)
1/4 cup Greek yogurt.

1 tablespoon of lime juice.

Method of preparation:

1. Season chicken: Rub the chicken breasts with olive oil, paprika, salt, and pepper.
2. Grill Chicken: Preheat a grill or grill pan to medium heat. Grill chicken for 6-7 minutes per side, or until thoroughly done. Let it rest for a few minutes before slicing.
3. Prepare Wrap: Spread Greek yogurt on each tortilla. Combine the cut chicken, avocado, mixed greens, and cherry tomatoes.
4. Wrap: Drizzle with lime juice, roll the tortillas, and serve.

Nutritional Value per Serving:

- Calories: 400.
- Protein: 30 grams.
- Carbohydrate: 38g
- Fat: 18g
- Fiber: 9 grams.

Serving Size: Four wraps.

Time for preparation: 30 minutes.

Lentil Soup With Vegetables

Ingredients:

1 cup green or brown lentils.

1 tablespoon of olive oil.

Chop one onion and cut two cloves of garlic.

Dice two carrots and two celery stalks.

One zucchini, diced

1 can (14 ounces) Diced tomatoes

4 cups veggie broth.

1 teaspoon cumin.

1/2 teaspoon turmeric.

Add salt and pepper to taste.

2 cups of fresh spinach.

Method of preparation:

1. Sauté vegetables. In a large saucepan, heat the olive oil over medium heat. Sauté onion, garlic, carrots, and celery until softened.

2. Mix in the lentils, diced tomatoes, vegetable broth, cumin, turmeric, salt, and pepper. Bring to a boil.

3. Simmer Soup: Reduce heat to low, cover, and cook for 30 minutes, or until lentils are cooked.

4. Finish by adding the zucchini and spinach, simmering for another 5 minutes until the zucchini is soft. Adjust the seasoning as required.

Nutritional Value per Serving:

- Calories: 270
- Protein: 14 grams.
- Carbs: 44g
- Fat: 5g
- Fiber: 15 grams.

Serving Size: Six Servings

Time for preparation: 45 minutes

Spinach and Feta Stuffed Peppers

Ingredients:

4 huge bell peppers, any color.

1 tablespoon of olive oil.

1 onion, chopped

2 garlic cloves, minced

1 cup of cooked brown rice.

2 cups fresh spinach, chopped.

1/2 cup crumbled feta cheese.

1 teaspoon of oregano.

Add salt and pepper to taste.

Method of preparation:

- Prepare peppers: Preheat the oven to 375° Fahrenheit (190° Celsius). Cut the pepper tops off and remove the seeds and membranes.
- Sauté Filling: Heat olive oil in a skillet over medium heat. Add the onion and garlic and sauté until transparent. Stir in the spinach until wilted.
- Mix Filling: In a bowl, combine cooked rice, spinach combination, feta cheese, oregano, salt, and pepper.
- Stuff the peppers with the mixture and place in a roasting tray.
- Cover with foil and bake for 30 minutes. Remove the foil and bake for another 10 minutes.

Nutritional Value per Serving:

- Calories: 210, protein: 7g.
- Carbohydrate: 28 grams
- Fat: 9g
- Fiber: 5 grams.

Serving Size: Four stuffed peppers.

Time to Prepare: 50 minutes

Chickpea and Tomato Salad. Ingredients:

1 can (15 oz) of chickpeas, drained and rinsed

1 cup cherry tomatoes, halved

One cucumber, diced

1/4 cup red onion, finely chopped

1/4 cup fresh parsley, chopped

2 tablespoons of olive oil.

2 teaspoons of lemon juice.

Add salt and pepper to taste.

1/4 teaspoon of cumin (optional)

Method of preparation:

1. To make the salad, combine: In a large mixing basin, add chickpeas, cherry tomatoes, cucumber, red onion, and parsley.
2. Dress Salad: In a small bowl, combine olive oil, lemon juice, salt, pepper, and cumin.
3. Toss Salad: Toss the salad with the dressing until completely combined.
4. Chill: Refrigerate for at least 30 minutes before serving to let the flavors combine.

Nutritional Value per Serving:

- Calories: 240
- Protein: 8 grams.
- Carbs: 30g
- Fat: 11g
- Fiber: 9 grams.

Serving Size: Four servings.

Time for preparation: 15 minutes.

Dinner Recipes

Baked Salmon and Asparagus

Ingredients:
4 salmon fillets, approximately 6 oz each.
1 bunch asparagus, trimmed
2 tablespoons of olive oil.
Mince two garlic cloves and slice one lemon.
Add salt and pepper to taste.
Fresh dill (optional).
Method of preparation:
1. Preheat the Oven: Preheat the oven to 400 °F (200 °C).
2. Prepare the Baking Sheet: Cover a baking sheet with parchment paper or gently oil it.
3. Arrange Ingredients: Place salmon fillets on one side of the baking sheet, and asparagus on the other.
4. Season Salmon: Drizzle olive oil on fish and asparagus. Sprinkle with minced garlic, salt, pepper, and fresh dill, if desired.
5. Top the salmon with lemon wedges.
6. Bake for 15-18 minutes, or until the salmon flakes easily with a fork and the asparagus is soft.

Nutritional Value per Serving:
- Calories: 380
- Protein: 34 grams.
- Carbs: 6g
- Fat: 24g
- Fiber: 2 grams.

Serving Size: Four servings.

Time for preparation: 25 minutes.

Zucchini Noodles with Pesto and Cherry Tomatoes

Ingredients:
4 spiralized medium zucchinis.
1 cup cherry tomatoes, halved
1/4 cup basil pesto (store-bought or homemade).
2 tablespoons of olive oil.
1/4 cup shredded Parmesan cheese (optional)
Add salt and pepper to taste.

Method of preparation:
1. Prepare the zucchini: Spiralize zucchini to make noodles. Set aside.
2. Sauté tomatoes: In a large skillet, heat the olive oil over medium heat. Add the cherry tomatoes and simmer until they soften.
3. Zucchini Noodles: Sauté zucchini noodles in a pan until barely cooked, about 2-3 minutes.
4. Mix with pesto: Remove from heat and stir with pesto, salt, and pepper.
5. Sprinkle with Parmesan cheese before serving, if preferred.

Nutritional Value per Serving:
- Calories: 220
- Protein: 6 grams.
- Carbohydrate: 15 grams
- Fat: 18g
- Fiber: 4 grams.

Serving Size: Four servings.
Time for preparation: 15 minutes.

Grilled Lemon Herb Chicken

Ingredients:

4 boneless and skinless chicken breasts.

1/4 cup olive oil.

1/4 cup lemon juice.

3 garlic cloves, minced

1 teaspoon of dried oregano.

1 teaspoon dried thyme.

Add salt and pepper to taste.

Lemon wedges for serving.

Method of preparation:

1. Prepare marinade: In a bowl, combine the olive oil, lemon juice, garlic, oregano, thyme, salt, and pepper.
2. Marinate Chicken: Place the chicken breasts in a resealable bag and pour the marinade over them. Seal and chill for at least 30 minutes, ideally two hours.
3. Preheat Grill: Preheat the grill to medium-high.
4. Grill Chicken: Remove the chicken from the marinade and grill for 6-7 minutes on each side, or until thoroughly done.
5. Serve with lemon wedges.

Nutritional Value per Serving:

- Calories: 310 Protein: 36 grams
- Carbs: 2g
- Fat: 18g
- Fiber: 0 grams.

Serving Size: Four servings.

Time of preparation: 40 minutes (including marinating time).

Stuffed bell peppers with quinoa and turkey

Ingredients:
Four huge bell peppers.
1 tablespoon of olive oil.
1/2 onion, chopped.
2 garlic cloves, minced
1 pound of ground turkey.
1 cup cooked quinoa.
1 can (14 ounces) Diced tomatoes, drained
1 teaspoon cumin.
1 teaspoon of paprika.
Add salt and pepper to taste.
1 cup of shredded mozzarella cheese (optional).

Method of preparation:

1. Preheat the Oven: Preheat the oven to 375° Fahrenheit (190° Celsius).
2. Prepare peppers: Cut the pepper tops off and remove the seeds and membranes.
3. Cook Filling: In a pan, heat the olive oil over medium heat. Add the onion and garlic and sauté until transparent. Add the ground turkey and heat until browned. Stir in the quinoa, diced tomatoes, cumin, paprika, salt, and pepper.
4. Stuff the peppers with the turkey mixture and place in a baking tray.
5. Cover with foil and bake for 30 minutes. Remove the foil, sprinkle with cheese if desired, and bake for another 10 minutes.

Nutritional Value per Serving:

- Calories: 340
- Protein: 30 grams.

- Carbohydrate: 28 grams
- Fat: 14g
- Fiber: 6 grams.

Serving Size: Four stuffed peppers.
Time to Prepare: 50 minutes

Eggplant Parmesan (Baked)

Ingredients:

2 medium eggplants, cut into half-inch rounds

1 cup of whole wheat breadcrumbs.

1/2 cup of grated Parmesan cheese.

Two eggs, beaten

1 tablespoon of olive oil.

2 cups of marinara sauce.

1 cup shredded mozzarella cheese.

1 teaspoon dried basil.

Add salt and pepper to taste.

Method of preparation:

1. Preheat your oven to 375°F (190°C).
2. Prepare the Eggplant: Sprinkle salt over the eggplant slices and let aside for 15 minutes. Pat dry with paper towels.
3. Bread Eggplant: Combine breadcrumbs and Parmesan cheese in a shallow dish. Dip eggplant slices in beaten eggs, then coat with the breadcrumb mixture.
4. Bake Eggplant: Place on a baking sheet lined with parchment paper. Drizzle with olive oil, then bake for 20 minutes, turning halfway.

5. Assemble dish: In a baking dish, put a layer of marinara sauce. Layer the roasted eggplant with additional sauce and mozzarella cheese. Repeat layers, finishing with the cheese and basil on top.

6. Bake for 25-30 minutes, until bubbling and brown.

Nutritional Value per Serving:

- Calories: 360
- Protein: 18 g.
- Carbohydrate: 38g
- Fat: 16g
- Fiber: 10 grams.

Serving Size: Four servings.

Time for preparation: 60 minutes

These supper recipes are delicious and healthy, making them ideal for a gout-friendly diet. If you have any additional questions or need assistance, please do not hesitate to ask!

Snacks Recipes

Cucumber and Hummus Bites.

Ingredients:

1 big cucumber, cut into 1/4-inch rounds.

1 cup of hummus, either store-bought or homemade

1 tablespoon fresh dill, chopped.

1 tablespoon of olive oil.

Add salt and pepper to taste.

Optional toppings include cherry tomato halves, chopped olives, and red pepper flakes.

Method of preparation:

1. Prepare the Cucumber: Slice the cucumbers into rounds and place them on a serving plate.
2. Spread Hummus: Add a dollop of hummus to each cucumber slice.
3. Add toppings: Drizzle with olive oil and season with fresh dill, salt, and pepper. For more taste, add optional toppings like cherry tomatoes, olives, or red pepper flakes.
4. Serve immediately as a refreshing and crisp snack.

Nutritional Value per Serving:

- Calories: 100.
- Protein: 2 grams.
- Carbohydrate: 10 grams
- Fat: 6g
- Fiber: 3 grams.

Serving Size: 4 servings (about 12 nibbles).

Time of preparation: ten minutes.

Almond Butter with Apple Slices

Ingredients:

2 medium apples (e.g. Gala or Fuji), cored and sliced

1/4 cup almond butter.

One tablespoon honey (optional)

1 teaspoon of cinnamon (optional).

Method of preparation:

1. Slice apples: Core the apples and cut them into small wedges.
2. Prepare Almond Butter: In a small bowl, combine almond butter, honey, and cinnamon, if preferred.

3. Serve: Place apple slices on a platter and serve with a side of almond butter for dipping.

Nutritional Value per Serving:

- Calories: 210
- Protein: 4 grams.
- Carbs: 29g
- Fat: 11g
- Fiber: 6 grams.

Serving Size: Two servings

Time of preparation: 5 minutes.

Roasted chickpeas

Ingredients:

1 can (15 oz) of chickpeas, drained and rinsed

1 tablespoon of olive oil.

1 teaspoon of smoked paprika.

1/2 teaspoon of garlic powder.

1/2 teaspoon cumin.

Add salt and pepper to taste.

Method of preparation:

1. Preheat the Oven: Preheat the oven to 400 °F (200 °C).
2. Dry chickpeas: To remove extra moisture from chickpeas, pat them dry using paper towels.
3. Season chickpeas: In a bowl, combine the chickpeas, olive oil, smoked paprika, garlic powder, cumin, salt, and pepper.
4. Roast chickpeas: Spread the chickpeas in a single layer on a baking sheet. Roast for 25-30 minutes, stirring halfway through, or until crisp and golden.
5. Cool and Let it cool somewhat before serving as a crispy snack.

Nutritional Value per Serving:
- Calories: 180
- Protein: 6g.
- Carbohydrate: 24g
- Fat: 7g
- Fiber: 5 grams.

Serving Size: Four servings.

Time for preparation: 35 minutes.

Carrot sticks with Greek Yogurt Dip

Ingredients:

4 huge carrots peeled and sliced into sticks.

1 cup Greek yogurt.

1 tablespoon of lemon juice.

1 teaspoon dill weed, fresh or dried

Add salt and pepper to taste.

Method of preparation:

1. Prepare carrots: Peel and chop the carrots into sticks. Arrange on a serving dish.
2. Make dip: In a bowl, add Greek yogurt, lemon juice, dill weed, salt, and pepper.
3. Serve carrot sticks with a Greek yogurt dip.

Nutritional Value per Serving:
- Calories: 90.
- Protein: 6 grams.
- Carbohydrate: 15 grams
- Fat: 2g
- Fiber: 3 grams.

Serving Size: Four servings.

Time of preparation: ten minutes.

Mixed Nuts & Seeds Trail mix

Ingredients:
1/2 cup almonds.
1/2 cup walnuts.
1/4 cup pumpkin seeds.
1/4 cup sunflower seeds.
1/4 cup dried cranberries.
1/4 cup of dark chocolate chips (optional)
1 teaspoon of cinnamon (optional).

Method of preparation:
1. Combine ingredients: In a large mixing bowl, add almonds, walnuts, pumpkin seeds, sunflower seeds, dried cranberries, and chocolate chips.
2. Add Flavor: If desired, sprinkle with cinnamon and stir thoroughly.
3. Serve immediately, or keep in an airtight jar for up to two weeks.

Nutritional Value per Serving:
- Calories: 200.
- Protein: 5 grams.
- Carbohydrate: 16g
- Fat: 14g
- Fiber: 3 grams.

Serving Size: Four servings
Time of preparation: 5 minutes.

These snacks are healthy, quick to make, and ideal for anybody trying to follow a gout-friendly diet. Please let me know if you need any further information or recipes.

Dessert Recipes

Chia Seed Pudding with Berries

Ingredients:
1/4 cup of chia seeds
1 cup almond milk (or whatever milk you want)
1 tablespoon honey or maple syrup.
1 teaspoon of vanilla essence.
1/2 cup mixed berries (such as blueberries, strawberries, and raspberries).
Optional toppings include chopped almonds, coconut flakes, and granola.

Method of preparation:
1. Mix. Ingredients: In a dish or container, mix the chia seeds, almond milk, honey, and vanilla essence. Stir carefully to prevent clumps.
2. Refrigerate: Cover and chill for at least 4 hours, or overnight, until the pudding thickens.
3. Before serving, stir the pudding and garnish with mixed berries and optional toppings such as sliced almonds or coconut flakes.

Nutritional Value per Serving:
- Calories: 230
- Protein: 5 grams.
- Carbohydrate: 27 grams

- Fat: 11g
- Fiber: 11 grams.

Serving Size: Two servings

Time of preparation: 5 minutes (plus 4 hours of chilling time)

Baked pears with cinnamon and honey.

Ingredients:

4 ripe pears (halved and cored).

2 tablespoons of honey.

1 teaspoon ground cinnamon.

1/4 cup chopped walnuts.

1 tablespoon unsalted butter, melted.

Optional: Greek yogurt or vanilla ice cream to serve

Method of preparation:

1. Preheat the Oven: Preheat the oven to 350° Fahrenheit (175° Celsius).
2. Prepare the pears: Place the pear halves in a baking dish, cut side up.
3. Add toppings: Drizzle honey over pears, sprinkle with cinnamon, and top with chopped walnuts. Pour melted butter over top.
4. Bake for 25-30 minutes, or until the pears are soft and faintly caramelized.
5. Serve warm, with a dollop of Greek yogurt or vanilla ice cream, if preferred.

Nutritional Value per Serving:

- Calories: 180
- Protein: 2 grams.
- Carbs: 33g

- Fat: 7g
- Fiber: 5 grams.

Serving Size: Four servings
Time for preparation: 35 minutes.

Frozen Banana and Berry Sorbet.

Ingredients:

2 ripe bananas cut and frozen.

1 cup mixed frozen berries (such as strawberries, blueberries, and raspberries)

1 tablespoon honey or agave syrup (optional).

1 teaspoon of lemon juice.

Fresh mint leaves for garnish (optional).

Method of preparation:

1. Blend. Ingredients: In a food processor or blender, combine the frozen bananas, mixed berries, honey, and lemon juice. Blend until smooth and creamy.
2. Adjust sweetness: Taste and add more honey if necessary.
3. Serve by scooping into dishes and garnishing with fresh mint leaves, as preferred.

Nutritional Value per Serving:

- Calories: 120.
- Protein: 1 g.
- Carbs: 30g
- Fat: 0g
- Fiber: 5 grams.

Serving Size: Four servings
Time of preparation: Ten minutes.

Oatmeal Cookies with Raisins

Ingredients:

1 cup rolled oats.

1/2 cup of whole wheat flour.

1/2 cup raisins.

1/4 cup unsalted, softened butter

1/4 cup honey or brown sugar.

1 egg

1 teaspoon of vanilla essence.

1/2 teaspoon of baking powder.

Half a teaspoon of crushed cinnamon

1/4 teaspoon salt.

Method of Preparation:

1. Preheat the oven to 350° Fahrenheit (175° Celsius). Line a baking sheet with parchment paper.
2. Mix Wet. Ingredients: In a mixing dish, combine butter and honey. Add the egg and vanilla extract, and mix until smooth.
3. Dry ingredients: In a separate dish, mix oats, whole wheat flour, baking powder, cinnamon, and salt.
4. Form dough: Stir in the dry ingredients until well blended. Fold in raisins.
5. Shaped Cookies: Drop tablespoon-sized dough balls onto the prepared baking sheet, spaced equally apart.
6. Bake for 10 to 12 minutes, or until the sides turn golden brown.
7. Allow the cookies to cool on the baking sheet for a few minutes before moving them to a wire rack.

Nutritional Value per Serving:

- Calories: 110.
- Protein: 2 grams.

- Carbohydrate: 17g
- Fat: 4g
- Fiber: 2 grams.

Serving Size: 18 cookies.

Time to Prepare: 20 minutes

Apple & Walnut Crumble

Ingredients:

4 medium apples, peeled, cored and sliced.

1/2 cup chopped walnuts.

1/2 cup rolled oats.

1/4 cup whole wheat flour.

1/4 cup honey or maple syrup.

1/4 cup unsalted butter melted

1 teaspoon ground cinnamon.

1/2 teaspoon of ground nutmeg.

1/4 teaspoon salt.

Method of preparation:

1. Preheat the Oven: Preheat the oven to 350° Fahrenheit (175° Celsius).
2. Prepare apples: In a baking dish, evenly distribute the apple pieces.
3. Make Crumble Topping: In a mixing bowl, combine oats, whole wheat flour, walnuts, cinnamon, nutmeg, and salt. Mix in the honey and melted butter until it resembles coarse crumbs.
4. Sprinkle crumble mixture over apples.
5. Bake for 25-30 minutes, or until the apples are soft and the topping turns golden brown.

6. Serve warm, garnished with a scoop of vanilla ice cream or a dollop of whipped cream.

Nutritional Value per Serving:

- Calories: 250.
- Protein: 3 grams.
- Carbs: 39g
- Fat: 11g
- Fiber: 5 grams.

Serving Size: Six servings.

Time of preparation: 40 minutes.

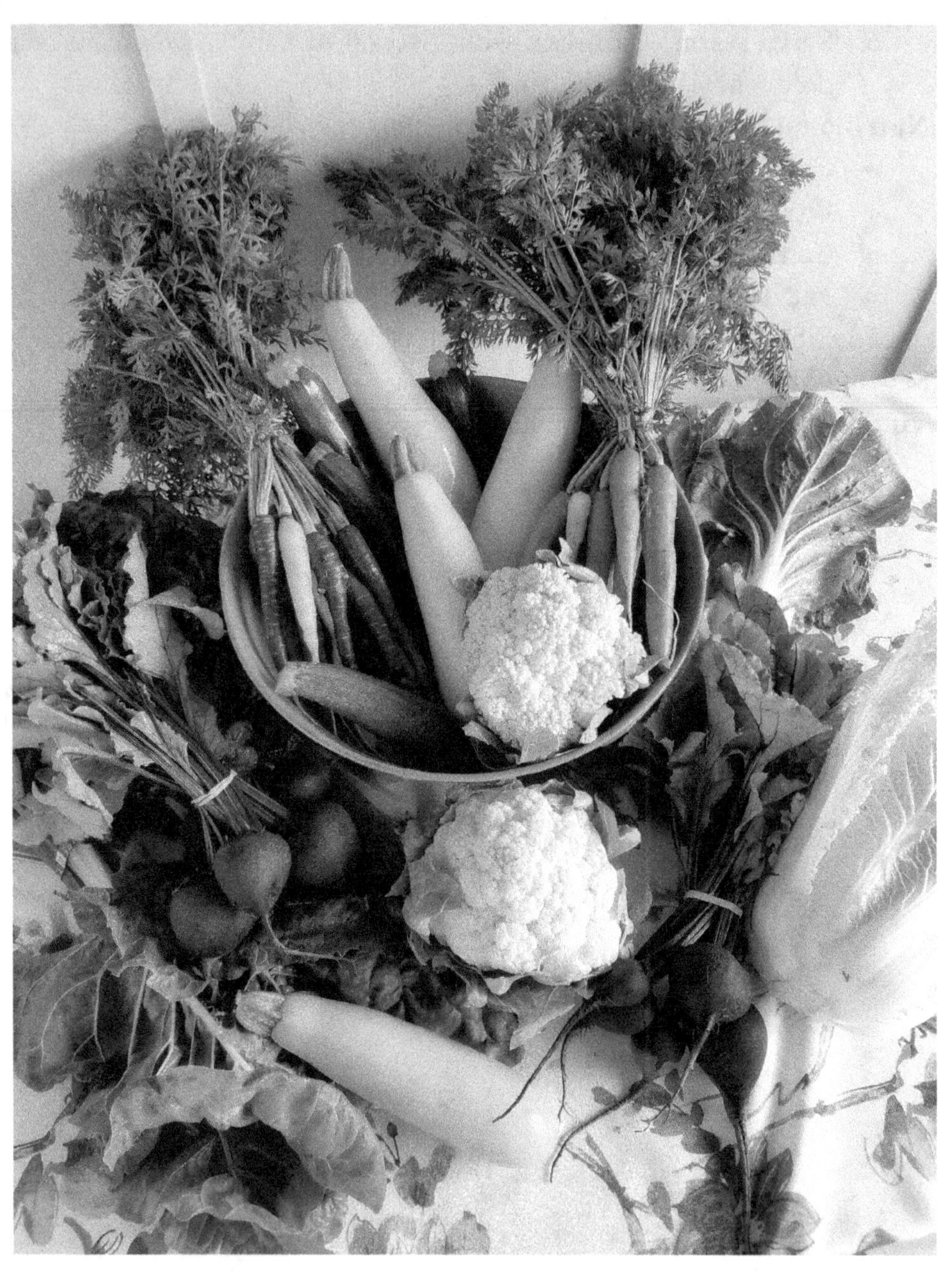

CHAPTER THREE

Creating a Gout-Friendly Meal Plan

Planning Balanced Meals for Gout Management

1. Include a Variety of Foods

Aim to include a variety of foods from all food groups in your meals to ensure you get a wide range of nutrients. Incorporate fruits, vegetables, whole grains, lean proteins, and low-fat dairy into your daily diet.

2. Choose Low-Purine Foods

Focus on selecting foods that are low in purines, as these can help reduce uric acid levels in the blood and minimize the risk of gout attacks. Good options include fruits, vegetables, whole grains, legumes, nuts, and seeds.

3. Emphasize Fruits and Vegetables

Fruits and vegetables are rich in vitamins, minerals, and antioxidants, and are low in purines, making them ideal choices for individuals with gout. Aim to fill half of your plate with fruits and vegetables at each meal to maximize nutrient intake and support gout management.

4. Incorporate Whole Grains

Whole grains, such as brown rice, quinoa, oats, barley, and whole wheat bread, are high in fiber and nutrients and can help promote satiety and stabilize blood sugar levels. Choose whole grains over refined grains to support overall health and gout management.

5. Opt for Lean Proteins

Choose lean sources of protein, such as poultry, fish, tofu, tempeh, and legumes, instead of high-purine meats like red meat and organ meats. These protein sources are lower in purines and can provide essential nutrients without increasing the risk of gout attacks.

6. Include Healthy Fats

Incorporate sources of healthy fats into your meals, such as avocados, nuts, seeds, and olive oil. These fats are rich in omega-3 fatty acids and monounsaturated fats, which have anti-inflammatory properties and can help reduce inflammation associated with gout.

7. Watch Portion Sizes

Pay attention to portion sizes to avoid overeating, especially high-purine foods. Eating large portions of high-purine foods can increase uric acid levels in the blood and trigger gout attacks. Use smaller plates, measure serving sizes, and practice mindful eating to prevent overconsumption.

8. Stay Hydrated

Drink plenty of water throughout the day to stay hydrated and support uric acid excretion. Aim for at least 8-10 cups of water per day, and limit intake of sugary beverages and alcohol, which can contribute to dehydration and increase the risk of gout attacks.

9. Plan Ahead

Take time to plan your meals and snacks in advance to ensure you have nutritious options readily available. Stock your kitchen with healthy ingredients, prepare meals in batches, and pack portable snacks to take with you when you're on the go.

10. Listen to Your Body

Pay attention to how different foods affect your body and adjust your diet accordingly. Keep a food diary to track your intake and any symptoms you experience, and consult with a registered dietitian or healthcare provider for personalized guidance and recommendations.

By planning balanced meals that include a variety of nutrient-rich foods and emphasize low-purine options, individuals with gout can effectively manage their symptoms and reduce the frequency of gout attacks. With careful meal planning and dietary modifications, you can support your overall health and well-being while living well with gout.

Portion Control and Moderation for Gout Management

1. Understand Portion Sizes

Understanding appropriate portion sizes is key to managing your caloric intake and maintaining a healthy weight. Use visual cues, such as your hand or common household objects, to estimate portion sizes of different foods. For example, a serving of meat should be about the size of a deck of cards, and a serving of pasta should be about the size of a tennis ball.

2. Use Smaller Plates

Using smaller plates can help control portion sizes by reducing the amount of food you serve yourself. Choose plates that are 9-10 inches in diameter, rather than larger plates, to encourage smaller portions and prevent overeating.

3. Measure Serving Sizes

Use measuring cups, spoons, and kitchen scales to accurately measure serving sizes of foods, especially high-calorie and high-purine foods. This can help prevent overeating and ensure you're consuming appropriate portions to support your gout management goals.

4. Practice Mindful Eating

Practice mindful eating by paying attention to your hunger and fullness cues and eating slowly and attentively. Chew your food thoroughly, savoring each bite, and stop eating when you feel satisfied, rather than full. This can help prevent overeating and promote better digestion.

5. Fill Half Your Plate with Fruits and Vegetables

Fruits and vegetables are low in calories and high in fiber and nutrients, making them ideal choices for filling up your plate without excess calories. Aim to fill half of your plate with fruits and vegetables at each meal to promote satiety and support gout management.

6. Limit High-Calorie and High-Purine Foods

High-calorie and high-purine foods, such as red meat, processed foods, sugary snacks, and alcoholic beverages, should be consumed in moderation to prevent excessive calorie and purine intake. Enjoy these foods occasionally and in small portions to minimize their impact on gout symptoms.

7. Practice the Plate Method

Use the plate method as a guide for creating balanced meals that include appropriate portion sizes of different food groups. Divide your plate into sections, half filled with fruits and vegetables, a quarter with lean protein, and a quarter with whole grains or starchy vegetables.

8. Listen to Your Body

Pay attention to how different foods affect your body and adjust your portion sizes accordingly. Notice how certain foods make you feel and whether they trigger gout symptoms. Use this information to make informed decisions about portion sizes and food choices that support your gout management goals.

9. Plan Ahead

Plan your meals and snacks in advance to ensure you have nutritious options readily available and avoid compulsive eating. Prepare healthy meals in advance, portion out snacks into individual servings, and pack portable snacks to take with you when you're on the go.

10. Seek Support and Accountability

Enlist the support of friends, family members, or a healthcare provider to help you stay accountable to your portion control and moderation goals. Share your goals with others, seek encouragement and support, and celebrate your progress along the way.

By practicing portion control and moderation, you can manage your caloric intake, maintain a healthy weight, and support your gout management efforts. With mindful eating habits and informed food choices, you can enjoy a balanced and satisfying diet while minimizing the risk of gout attacks and promoting overall health and well-being.

Hydration and Gout Management

1. Importance of Hydration

Staying hydrated is essential for managing gout, as adequate hydration helps to dilute uric acid in the blood and promote its excretion through urine. When you're well-hydrated, uric acid is more likely to be dissolved in the urine and flushed out of the body, reducing the risk of urate crystal formation in the joints.

2. Recommended Fluid Intake

Aim to drink plenty of fluids throughout the day to maintain hydration and support gout management. The Institute of Medicine recommends that men consume about 3.7 liters (125 ounces) of fluids per day and women consume about 2.7 liters (91 ounces) of fluids per day from all beverages and foods.

3. Water is Best

Water is the best choice for staying hydrated, as it contains no calories, sugar, or purines. Drinking water throughout the day can help prevent dehydration and promote optimal kidney function, which is crucial for uric acid excretion. Carry a reusable water bottle with you and sip on water regularly to stay hydrated.

4. Limit Sugary Beverages

Limit intake of sugary beverages, such as soda, fruit juice, and sweetened teas, as they can contribute to weight gain and increase the risk of gout attacks. These beverages provide empty calories and can lead to dehydration, both of which can exacerbate gout symptoms.

5. Watch Alcohol Consumption

Moderate alcohol consumption, particularly beer and liquor, can increase uric acid levels in the blood and trigger gout attacks. If you drink alcohol, do so in moderation and opt for lower-purine options, such as wine. Be sure to stay hydrated by drinking water alongside alcoholic beverages and limit intake to reduce the risk of gout flares.

6. Monitor Urine Output

Pay attention to your urine output and aim for pale yellow urine, which is a sign of adequate hydration. Dark yellow or amber-colored urine may indicate dehydration and insufficient fluid intake. If you're not urinating regularly or your urine is concentrated, drink more fluids to stay hydrated.

7. Hydration Tips

Drink water first thing in the morning and throughout the day to replenish fluids lost overnight and maintain hydration.

Carry a reusable water bottle with you and sip on water regularly, especially in hot weather or during physical activity.

Eat water-rich foods, such as fruits and vegetables, which can contribute to your overall fluid intake and support hydration.

Flavor water with fresh fruit slices or herbs, such as lemon, lime, cucumber, or mint, to enhance taste without adding calories or sugar.

8. Seek Medical Advice

If you have kidney problems or other medical conditions that affect fluid balance, consult with your healthcare provider for personalized hydration recommendations. They can help you determine the appropriate fluid intake for your individual needs and medical history.

By staying hydrated and maintaining adequate fluid intake, individuals with gout can help reduce the risk of gout attacks and support overall health and well-being. Incorporating hydration into your daily routine and making water your beverage of choice can contribute to effective gout management and improved quality of life.

Meal Planning Tips for Beginners

1. Set Realistic Goals

Start by setting realistic goals for your meal planning journey. Consider your schedule, cooking abilities, and dietary preferences, and set achievable objectives that you can stick to in the long term.

2. Create a Weekly Menu

Plan your meals for the week ahead by creating a weekly menu. Take into account breakfast, lunch, dinner, and snacks, and aim for a balance of nutrients and variety in your meals.

3. Consider Dietary Needs

Take into consideration any dietary restrictions or preferences when planning your meals. Whether you're vegetarian, vegan, gluten-free, or following a specific diet plan, tailor your meal plan to meet your individual needs.

4. Make a Shopping List

Once you've planned your meals for the week, create a shopping list of the ingredients you'll need. Check your pantry and fridge to see what items you already have on hand and prioritize purchasing fresh produce and perishable items.

5. Shop Smart

When grocery shopping, stick to your list and avoid impulse purchases. Choose fresh, whole foods whenever possible, and opt for seasonal produce to save money and enjoy peak flavor and nutrition.

6. Prep Ingredients in Advance

Spend some time prepping ingredients in advance to streamline the cooking process during the week. Wash and chop fruits and vegetables, marinate proteins, and cook grains or legumes ahead of time to save time and effort later.

7. Batch Cook

Consider batch cooking certain meals or components of meals to save time and ensure you have nutritious options readily available throughout the week. Cook large batches of soups, stews, casseroles, or grains and portion them out for easy meals or lunches.

8. Use Leftovers Creatively

Get creative with leftovers by repurposing them into new meals. For example, leftover roasted vegetables can be added to salads, sandwiches, or grain bowls, and cooked chicken can be used in wraps, stir-fries, or soups.

9. Keep It Simple

Don't feel pressured to make elaborate meals every night. Focus on simple, nourishing dishes that are easy to prepare and enjoy. Consider one-pot meals, sheet pan dinners, or slow cooker recipes for minimal cleanup and maximum flavor.

10. Be Flexible

Be flexible with your meal plan and adapt it as needed based on changes in your schedule, cravings, or ingredient availability. Don't be afraid to swap out recipes, improvise with ingredients, or dine out occasionally if it makes sense for you.

11. Embrace Variety

Incorporate variety into your meal plan by trying new recipes, cuisines, and ingredients. Experiment with different flavors, textures, and cooking techniques to keep meals interesting and enjoyable.

12. Practice Self-Care

Lastly, prioritize self-care and listen to your body's hunger and fullness cues. Make time for regular meals and snacks, and aim for a balanced diet that nourishes your body and supports your overall health and well-being.

By following these meal planning tips for beginners, you can streamline your meal preparation process, save time and money, and enjoy delicious and nutritious meals throughout the week. With practice and consistency, meal planning will become a valuable skill that helps you maintain a healthy lifestyle and reach your wellness goals.

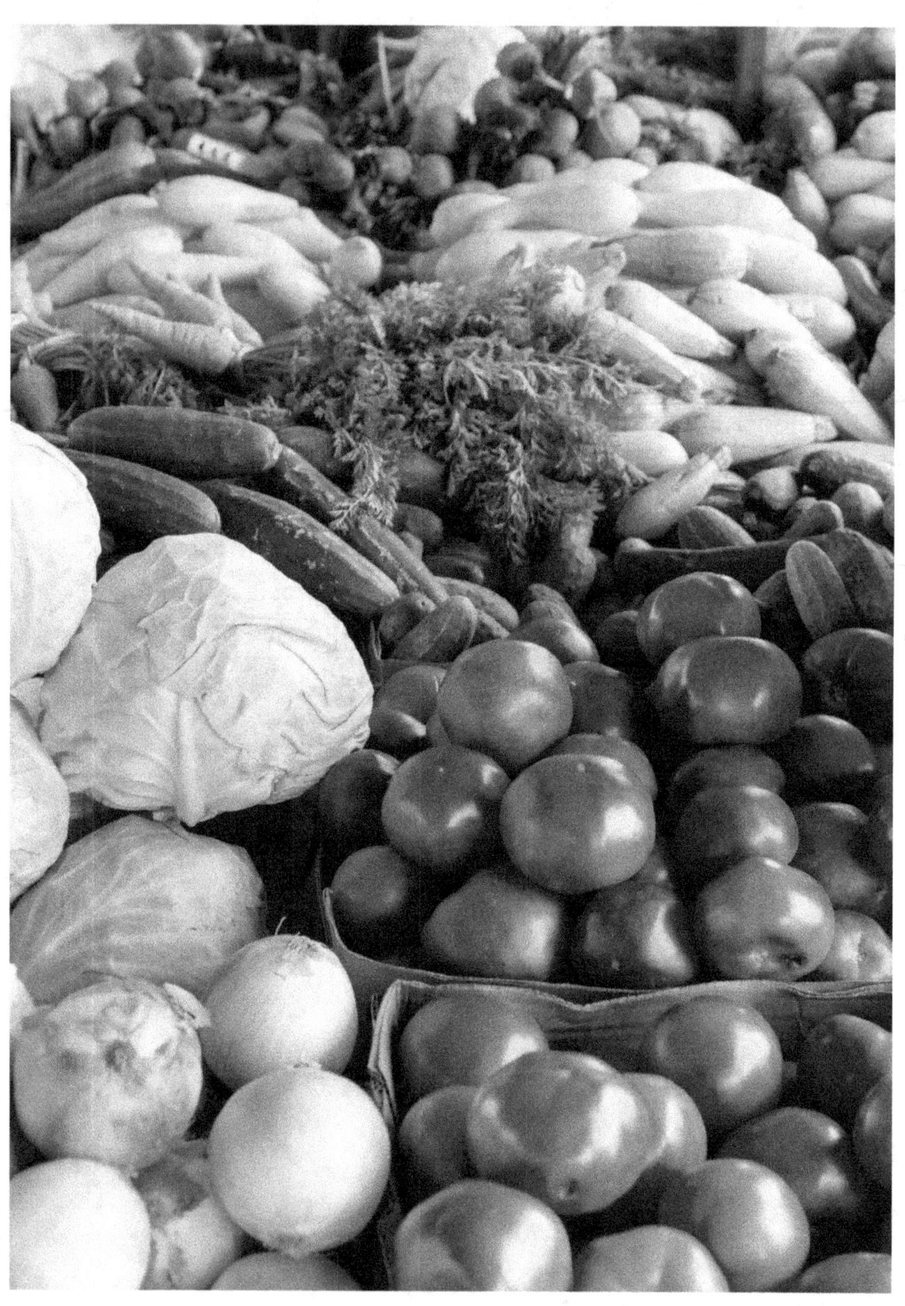

CHAPTER FOUR

Lifestyle Tips for Managing Gout

Exercise and Physical Activity for Gout Management

1. Importance of Exercise

Regular exercise is an essential component of gout management, as it can help reduce inflammation, improve joint function, and support overall health and well-being. Engaging in regular physical activity can also help maintain a healthy weight, which is important for managing gout symptoms.

2. Choose Low-Impact Activities

When selecting exercises, choose low-impact activities that are gentle on the joints, such as walking, swimming, cycling, or yoga. These activities can help improve cardiovascular fitness, strengthen muscles, and increase flexibility without putting excessive strain on the joints.

3. Start Slowly

If you're new to exercise or have been inactive for a while, start slowly and gradually increase the intensity and duration of your workouts over time. Begin with short sessions of low-intensity exercise and gradually build up to longer sessions or more challenging activities as your fitness improves.

4. Incorporate Strength Training

Include strength training exercises in your workout routine to build and maintain muscle mass, improve joint stability, and support overall joint health. Use resistance bands, free weights, or bodyweight exercises to target major muscle groups and strengthen the muscles surrounding the joints affected by gout.

5. Stretch Regularly

Incorporate stretching exercises into your routine to improve flexibility, reduce stiffness, and prevent injury. Focus on stretching the muscles and joints of the lower body, including the ankles, knees, hips, and lower back, which are commonly affected by gout.

6. Listen to Your Body

Pay attention to how your body responds to exercise and adjust your workout routine accordingly. If you experience pain, swelling, or discomfort during or after exercise, modify your activities or take a break to rest and recover. Consult with your healthcare provider if you have concerns about exercising with gout or other medical conditions.

7. Stay Hydrated

Drink plenty of water before, during, and after exercise to stay hydrated and support uric acid excretion. Adequate hydration is essential for maintaining joint health and preventing dehydration, which can exacerbate gout symptoms.

8. Warm Up and Cool Down

Always warm up before exercise with gentle movements and dynamic stretches to prepare your muscles and joints for activity. Similarly, cool down after exercise with static stretches to help relax and lengthen the muscles and reduce post-exercise stiffness.

9. Be Consistent

Make exercise a regular part of your routine by scheduling regular workouts and staying committed to your fitness goals. Aim for at least 150 minutes of moderate-intensity aerobic activity or 75 minutes of vigorous-intensity aerobic activity per week, as recommended by the Centers for Disease Control and Prevention (CDC).

10. Have Fun

Choose activities that you enjoy and that fit your interests, preferences, and lifestyle. Whether it's dancing, gardening, hiking, or playing a sport, finding activities that you love can make exercise more enjoyable and sustainable in the long term.

By incorporating regular exercise and physical activity into your routine, you can improve joint health, reduce inflammation, and support overall gout management. Be sure to consult with your healthcare provider before starting any new exercise program, especially if you have underlying health conditions or concerns about exercising with gout.

Weight Management for Gout

1. Importance of Weight Management

Maintaining a healthy weight is essential for managing gout, as excess body weight can contribute to elevated uric acid levels in the blood and increase the risk of gout attacks. Losing weight can help reduce the frequency and severity of gout symptoms and improve overall joint health and mobility.

2. Set Realistic Goals

Set realistic weight loss goals based on your current weight, health status, and personal preferences. Aim to lose weight gradually at a rate of 1-2 pounds per week, which is considered safe and sustainable for long-term weight management.

3. Adopt a Balanced Diet

Focus on adopting a balanced diet that includes a variety of nutrient-rich foods from all food groups. Choose whole grains, fruits, vegetables, lean proteins, and low-fat dairy products, and limit intake of high-calorie and high-fat foods. Pay attention to portion sizes and practice mindful eating to avoid overeating and support weight management.

4. Monitor Caloric Intake

Keep track of your daily caloric intake and aim to create a calorie deficit by consuming fewer calories than you expend through physical activity and metabolic processes. Use food journals or mobile apps to track your intake and make adjustments as needed to achieve your weight loss goals.

5. Increase Physical Activity

Incorporate regular physical activity into your routine to support weight loss and improve overall health. Aim for at least 150 minutes of moderate-intensity aerobic activity or 75 minutes of vigorous-intensity aerobic activity per week, as recommended by health authorities. Include a combination of cardiovascular exercise, strength training, and flexibility exercises to maximize calorie burn and support muscle maintenance.

6. Focus on Lifestyle Changes

Instead of relying on fad diets or quick-fix solutions, focus on making sustainable lifestyle changes that promote long-term weight management. Adopt healthy eating habits, such as cooking at home, planning meals in advance, and practicing portion control. Make physical activity a regular part of your routine and find activities that you enjoy and can stick to in the long term.

7. Seek Support

Enlist the support of friends, family members, or a healthcare provider to help you stay accountable to your weight loss goals. Consider joining a support group or working with a registered dietitian or certified personal trainer for personalized guidance and encouragement.

8. Be Patient and Persistent

Weight loss takes time and effort, so be patient and persistent in your efforts to reach your goals. Celebrate your progress along the way, even small victories, and don't get discouraged by setbacks or plateaus. Stay focused on your long-term health and well-being and continue making positive lifestyle changes.

9. Address Underlying Factors

If you're struggling to lose weight despite making healthy lifestyle changes, consider addressing underlying factors that may be contributing to weight gain, such as stress, sleep deprivation, or medication side effects. Talk to your healthcare provider for personalized recommendations and support.

10. Monitor Progress and Adjust Goals

Regularly monitor your progress towards your weight loss goals and adjust your strategies as needed to stay on track. Track your weight, body measurements, and other indicators of progress, and celebrate your achievements along the way. Be flexible and willing to modify your goals and strategies based on your changing needs and circumstances.

By focusing on weight management through a combination of healthy eating, regular physical activity, and lifestyle changes, individuals with gout can improve their overall health and reduce the frequency and severity of gout attacks. Be patient, stay consistent, and prioritize your long-term well-being as you work towards achieving and maintaining a healthy weight.

Stress Management for Gout

1. Understand the Connection

Stress can exacerbate gout symptoms by triggering inflammation and increasing pain perception. Understanding the connection between stress and gout can help you develop effective strategies for managing stress and minimizing its impact on your symptoms.

2. Identify Stress Triggers

Identify the specific stressors in your life that contribute to feelings of tension, anxiety, or overwhelm. These may include work-related pressures, relationship issues, financial worries, or health concerns. By pinpointing your stress triggers, you can better anticipate and manage stressful situations.

3. Practice Relaxation Techniques

Incorporate relaxation techniques into your daily routine to help reduce stress and promote a sense of calm and well-being. Techniques such as deep breathing exercises, progressive muscle relaxation, mindfulness meditation, and guided imagery can help lower stress levels and improve overall mental and physical health.

4. Stay Active

Regular physical activity can help reduce stress and improve mood by promoting the release of endorphins, which are natural mood-boosting chemicals in the brain. Engage in activities that you enjoy, such as walking, swimming, yoga, or dancing, and make exercise a regular part of your routine to manage stress effectively.

5. Prioritize Self-Care

Prioritize self-care activities that promote relaxation, rejuvenation, and self-nurturing. Make time for hobbies, interests, and activities that bring you joy and fulfillment, whether it's reading, gardening, listening to music, or spending time in nature. Taking care of your physical, emotional, and mental well-being is essential for managing stress and supporting overall health.

6. Maintain a Healthy Lifestyle

Adopt a healthy lifestyle that supports stress management and overall well-being. Eat a balanced diet, get regular exercise, prioritize sleep, and limit intake of caffeine, alcohol, and nicotine, which can exacerbate stress and anxiety. Taking care of your physical health can help build resilience to stress and improve your ability to cope with life's challenges.

7. Build a Support System

Surround yourself with supportive friends, family members, and healthcare professionals who can provide encouragement, guidance, and practical assistance during times of stress. Having a strong support system can help you feel less isolated and more capable of coping with stressors effectively.

8. Practice Time Management

Manage your time effectively by prioritizing tasks, setting realistic goals, and breaking projects down into smaller, manageable steps. Use organizational tools, such as planners, calendars, or smartphone apps, to schedule activities, track deadlines, and stay on top of your responsibilities. By managing your time efficiently, you can reduce feelings of overwhelm and stress.

9. Seek Professional Help if Needed

If you're struggling to manage stress on your own, don't hesitate to seek professional help from a therapist, counselor, or mental health professional. They can provide support, guidance, and evidence-based techniques for managing stress and improving coping skills.

10. Practice Mindfulness

Cultivate mindfulness, or the practice of being present and fully engaged in the moment, as a way to reduce stress and increase resilience. Mindfulness techniques, such as mindful breathing, body scans, and mindful eating, can help you stay grounded, calm, and focused amidst life's challenges.

By incorporating stress management techniques into your daily routine, you can reduce the impact of stress on your gout symptoms and improve your overall quality of life. Experiment with different strategies to find what works best for you, and don't hesitate to reach out for support when needed. Taking proactive steps to manage stress can help you feel more empowered and resilient in the face of life's challenges.

Alcohol and Gout

1. Understand the Connection

Alcohol consumption is strongly linked to the development and exacerbation of gout. Alcohol can increase uric acid levels in the blood by promoting its production and impairing its excretion, leading to the formation of urate crystals in the joints and triggering gout attacks.

2. Know Your Limits

If you have gout, it's important to know your limits when it comes to alcohol consumption. While moderate alcohol consumption may not necessarily trigger gout attacks in everyone, excessive or frequent drinking can significantly increase the risk of gout flares.

3. Limit Intake of High-Purine Alcohols

Certain types of alcohol are higher in purines, compounds that break down into uric acid in the body, and can increase the risk of gout attacks. Beer, in particular, is associated with a higher risk of gout due to its high purine content, followed by liquor and wine. If you choose to drink alcohol, opt for lower-purine options, such as clear spirits like vodka or gin, and limit consumption of beer and liquor.

4. Hydrate Adequately

Drinking alcohol can lead to dehydration, which can exacerbate gout symptoms by reducing the excretion of uric acid from the body. To mitigate this effect, be sure to hydrate adequately by drinking plenty of water before, during, and after consuming alcohol. Aim to drink at least one glass of water for every alcoholic beverage consumed to stay hydrated and support uric acid excretion.

5. Moderation is Key

Moderation is key when it comes to alcohol consumption for individuals with gout. The Centers for Disease Control and Prevention (CDC) defines moderate alcohol consumption as up to one drink per day for women and up to two drinks per day for men. Exceeding these limits can increase the risk of gout attacks and other health problems.

6. Monitor Your Symptoms

Pay attention to how alcohol affects your gout symptoms and be mindful of any triggers or patterns. If you notice that certain types of alcohol or drinking habits consistently lead to gout flares, consider reducing or eliminating alcohol from your diet to help manage your symptoms more effectively.

7. Consider Lifestyle Changes

If you find it challenging to moderate your alcohol intake or experience frequent gout attacks despite limiting alcohol consumption, consider making lifestyle changes to support gout management. Focus on maintaining a healthy weight, following a balanced diet low in purines, staying hydrated, and engaging in regular physical activity to reduce the frequency and severity of gout flares.

8. Talk to Your Healthcare Provider

If you have questions or concerns about alcohol and its impact on your gout, don't hesitate to talk to your healthcare provider. They can provide personalized recommendations based on your individual health status, medication use, and lifestyle factors, and help you develop strategies for managing gout effectively.

9. Be Mindful of Triggers

In addition to alcohol, be mindful of other potential triggers for gout attacks, such as certain foods, medications, and lifestyle factors. Keep track of your symptoms and any factors that may contribute to gout flares, and make adjustments to your diet and lifestyle as needed to minimize the risk of future attacks.

10. Focus on Overall Health

Ultimately, focus on improving your overall health and well-being to better manage gout and reduce the impact of alcohol on your symptoms. Adopting healthy lifestyle habits, such as eating a balanced diet, staying active, managing stress, and getting adequate sleep, can help support gout management and promote optimal health in the long term.

By being mindful of your alcohol consumption and its impact on your gout symptoms, you can make informed choices that support your overall health and well-being. Remember to prioritize moderation, hydration, and lifestyle changes to effectively manage gout and reduce the risk of gout attacks.

Smoking and Gout

1. Understanding the Link

Smoking is not only harmful to overall health but can also exacerbate gout symptoms and increase the risk of gout attacks. Smoking is associated with higher levels of uric acid in the blood, as well as increased inflammation and oxidative stress, which can contribute to the development and progression of gout.

2. Increased Uric Acid Levels

Smoking has been shown to increase uric acid levels in the blood, which is a key factor in the development of gout. Elevated uric acid levels can lead to the formation of urate crystals in the joints, causing inflammation, pain, and swelling characteristic of gout attacks.

3. Reduced Uric Acid Excretion

Smoking can impair the kidneys' ability to excrete uric acid from the body, further contributing to elevated uric acid levels and the risk of gout attacks. This can lead to a vicious cycle of increased uric acid production and decreased uric acid excretion, making it more difficult to manage gout symptoms effectively.

4. Increased Inflammation

Smoking is a known inflammatory trigger and can exacerbate inflammation in the body, including in the joints affected by gout. Chronic inflammation can worsen gout symptoms and increase the frequency and severity of gout attacks, making it more challenging to manage the condition.

5. Impact on Treatment Efficacy

Smoking can also interfere with the effectiveness of medications used to manage gout, such as urate-lowering drugs (e.g., allopurinol, febuxostat). Studies have shown that smokers may have a poorer response to these medications compared to non-smokers, potentially leading to suboptimal gout management and increased disease burden.

6. Compounding Health Risks

In addition to its impact on gout, smoking is associated with a myriad of other health risks, including cardiovascular disease, respiratory problems, cancer, and premature death. Individuals with gout who smoke may face compounded health risks and a higher overall disease burden.

7. Quitting Smoking

Quitting smoking is one of the most important steps individuals with gout can take to improve their health and reduce the risk of gout attacks. Quitting smoking can lead to lower uric acid levels, reduced inflammation, and improved response to gout medications, ultimately helping to better manage gout symptoms and reduce disease progression.

8. Support Resources

If you're ready to quit smoking, there are many resources and support systems available to help you succeed. Consider reaching out to your healthcare provider for personalized guidance and treatment options, joining a smoking cessation program or support group, or using nicotine replacement therapies or medications to aid in quitting.

9. Focus on Healthy Habits

In addition to quitting smoking, focus on adopting other healthy habits that support gout management and overall well-being. Eat a balanced diet low in purines, maintain a healthy weight, stay physically active, manage stress, and avoid excessive alcohol consumption to reduce the risk of gout attacks and improve overall health.

10. Seek Professional Help

If you're struggling to quit smoking or have concerns about its impact on your gout, don't hesitate to seek professional help from your healthcare provider or a specialist in smoking cessation. They can provide personalized recommendations, support, and resources to help you quit smoking successfully and improve your overall health outcomes.

By quitting smoking and adopting a healthy lifestyle, individuals with gout can reduce inflammation, lower uric acid levels, and improve their overall health and well-being. Quitting smoking is a critical step in effectively managing gout and reducing the risk of gout attacks, as well as improving long-term health outcomes.

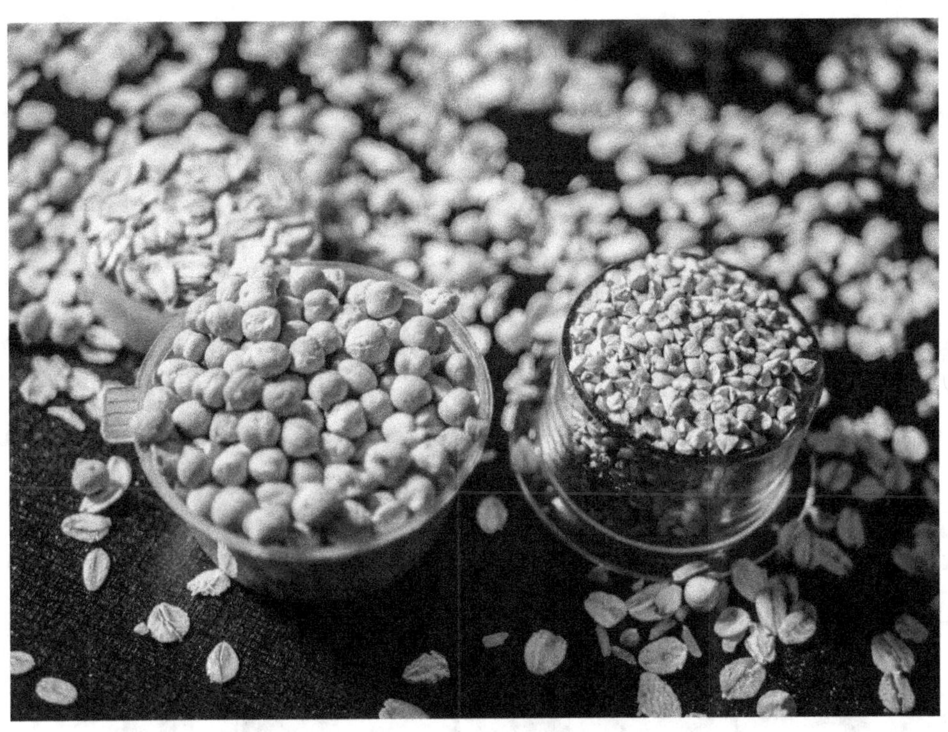

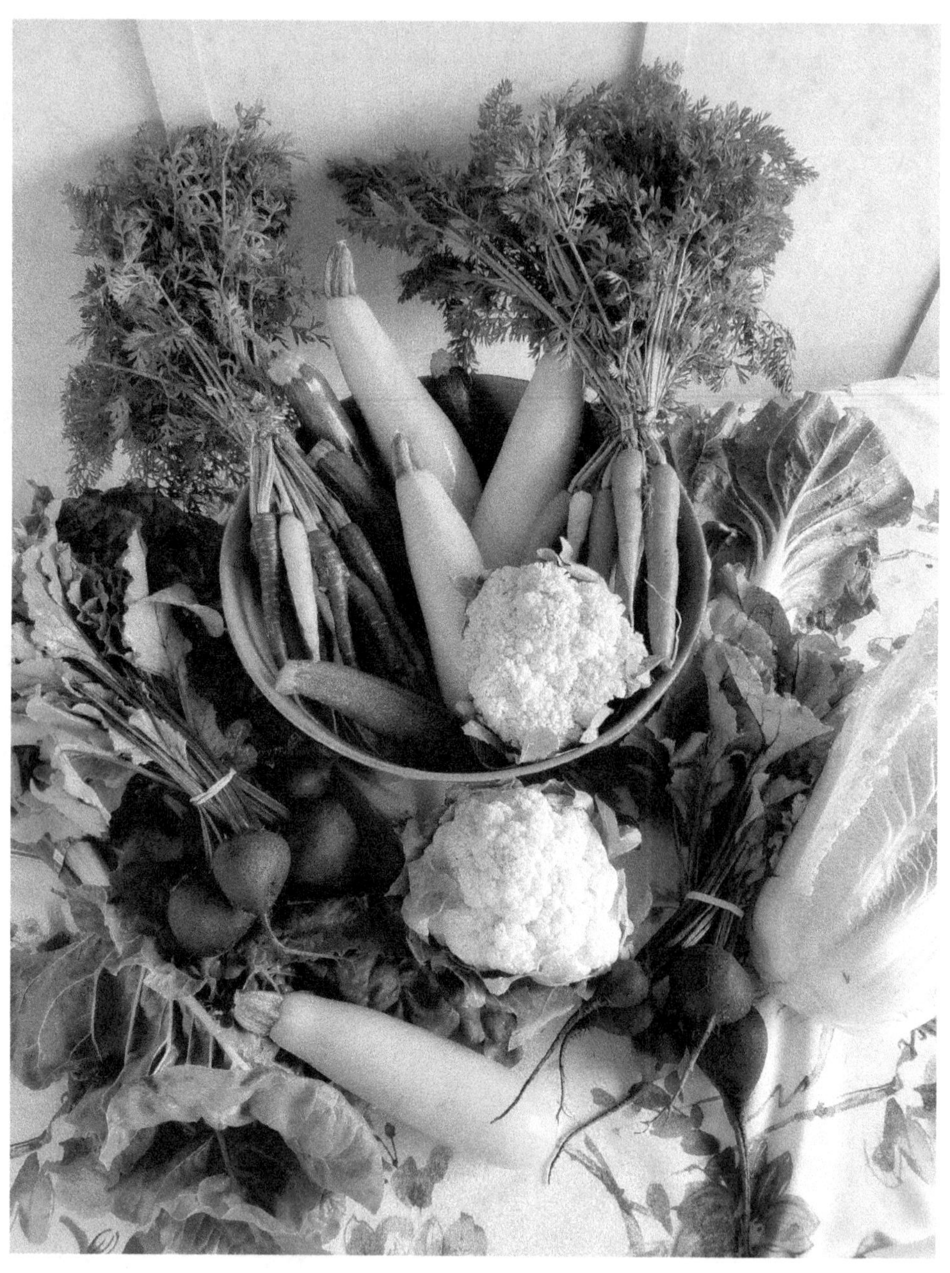

CHAPTER FIVE

Supplements and Natural Remedies

Supplements for Gout Management

1. Vitamin C

Vitamin C is a water-soluble antioxidant that has been shown to reduce serum uric acid levels by increasing uric acid excretion in the urine. Studies have suggested that supplementing with vitamin C may help lower the risk of gout attacks and reduce the severity of symptoms. Aim for a daily dose of 500-1000 milligrams of vitamin C to support gout management.

2. Cherry Extract

Cherry extract, derived from tart cherries, is rich in antioxidants and anti-inflammatory compounds known as anthocyanins. Research has shown that cherry extract supplementation may help reduce the frequency and severity of gout attacks by lowering serum uric acid levels and reducing inflammation. Consider taking cherry extract supplements or incorporating fresh or frozen cherries into your diet to support gout management.

3. Fish Oil/Omega-3 Fatty Acids

Fish oil supplements, which are high in omega-3 fatty acids, have anti-inflammatory properties that may benefit individuals with gout. Omega-3 fatty acids can help reduce inflammation in the body, which may help alleviate gout symptoms and lower the risk of gout attacks. Consider taking fish oil supplements or consuming fatty fish rich in omega-3s, such as salmon, mackerel, or sardines, to support gout management.

4. Bromelain

Bromelain is a mixture of enzymes found in pineapple that has anti-inflammatory properties. Studies have suggested that bromelain supplementation may help reduce inflammation and pain associated with gout attacks by inhibiting inflammatory pathways in the body. Consider taking bromelain supplements or incorporating fresh pineapple into your diet to support gout management.

5. Probiotics

Probiotics are beneficial bacteria that support gut health and immune function. Emerging research suggests that probiotic supplementation may help reduce inflammation and improve metabolic health, which could benefit individuals with gout. Consider taking a high-quality probiotic supplement containing a variety of strains to support gut health and overall well-being.

6. Turmeric/Curcumin

Turmeric is a spice that contains curcumin, a compound with powerful anti-inflammatory and antioxidant properties. Research has shown that curcumin supplementation may help reduce inflammation and pain associated with gout attacks by inhibiting inflammatory pathways in the body. Consider taking turmeric or curcumin supplements to support gout management.

7. Vitamin D

Vitamin D is important for bone health and immune function and may play a role in reducing inflammation in the body. Some studies have suggested that vitamin D deficiency may be associated with an increased risk of gout. Consider taking vitamin D supplements or getting adequate sun exposure to maintain optimal vitamin D levels and support gout management.

8. Quercetin

Quercetin is a flavonoid found in many fruits and vegetables with antioxidant and anti-inflammatory properties. Research has shown that quercetin supplementation may help reduce inflammation and oxidative stress in the body, which could benefit individuals with gout. Consider taking quercetin supplements or increasing your intake of quercetin-rich foods, such as apples, onions, and leafy greens, to support gout management.

9. Magnesium

Magnesium is an essential mineral that plays a role in over 300 enzymatic reactions in the body, including those involved in inflammation and muscle function. Some studies have suggested that magnesium supplementation may help reduce inflammation and lower the risk of gout attacks. Consider taking magnesium supplements or increasing your intake of magnesium-rich foods, such as leafy greens, nuts, seeds, and whole grains, to support gout management.

10. Always Consult Your Healthcare Provider

Before starting any new supplements or making significant changes to your diet or lifestyle, it's important to consult with your healthcare provider, especially if you have underlying health conditions or are taking medications. Your healthcare provider can help determine which supplements may be appropriate for you and provide personalized recommendations based on your individual health needs and goals.

Incorporating supplements into your gout management plan may help support overall health and reduce the frequency and severity of gout attacks. However, supplements should not be used as a substitute for medical treatment or lifestyle changes recommended by your healthcare provider. Be sure to discuss any questions or concerns with your healthcare provider before starting any new supplements.

Herbal Remedies for Gout and Their Efficacy

1. Devil's Claw (Harpagophytum procumbens)

Devil's claw is a plant native to southern Africa that has been traditionally used to treat inflammation and pain. Some studies suggest that devil's claw may have anti-inflammatory properties and could help reduce pain associated with gout attacks. However, more research is needed to confirm its efficacy and safety for gout management.

2. Turmeric (Curcuma longa)

Turmeric is a spice derived from the rhizomes of the Curcuma longa plant and contains curcumin, a compound with potent anti-inflammatory and antioxidant properties. Research has shown that curcumin may help reduce inflammation and pain associated with gout attacks by inhibiting inflammatory pathways in the body. Turmeric supplementation or consumption may be beneficial for individuals with gout, but more studies are needed to determine its effectiveness.

3. Ginger (Zingiber officinale)

Ginger is a popular spice with anti-inflammatory and analgesic properties that may help reduce pain and inflammation associated with gout attacks. Some studies have suggested that ginger supplementation or consumption may help alleviate gout symptoms, but more research is needed to confirm its efficacy and optimal dosage.

4. Celery Seed (Apium graveolens)

Celery seed is derived from the Apium graveolens plant and has been used in traditional medicine to treat inflammation and arthritis. Some studies have suggested that celery seed extract may help lower uric acid levels in the blood and reduce inflammation associated with gout attacks. However, more research is needed to determine its effectiveness and safety for gout management.

5. Cherry Extract

Cherry extract, derived from tart cherries, is rich in antioxidants and anti-inflammatory compounds known as anthocyanins. Research has shown that cherry extract supplementation may help reduce the frequency and severity of gout attacks by lowering serum uric acid levels and reducing inflammation. Consuming cherry extract or incorporating fresh or frozen cherries into the diet may be beneficial for individuals with gout.

6. Boswellia (Boswellia serrata)

Boswellia, also known as Indian frankincense, is a resin extracted from the Boswellia serrata tree and has been used in traditional medicine to treat inflammatory conditions. Some studies suggest that boswellia supplementation may help reduce inflammation and pain associated with gout attacks by inhibiting inflammatory pathways in the body. However, more research is needed to confirm its efficacy and safety for gout management.

7. Nettle Leaf (Urtica dioica)

Nettle leaf is derived from the Urtica dioica plant and has been used in traditional medicine to treat arthritis and other inflammatory conditions. Some studies have suggested that nettle leaf supplementation may help reduce inflammation and pain associated with gout attacks. However, more research is needed to determine its effectiveness and optimal dosage for gout management.

8. Bromelain

Bromelain is a mixture of enzymes found in pineapple that has anti-inflammatory properties. Research has shown that bromelain supplementation may help reduce inflammation and pain associated with gout attacks by inhibiting inflammatory pathways in the body. Consider taking bromelain supplements or incorporating fresh pineapple into the diet to support gout management.

9. Green Tea (Camellia sinensis)

Green tea is rich in antioxidants called catechins, which have anti-inflammatory and antioxidant properties. Some studies have suggested that green tea consumption may help reduce inflammation and lower uric acid levels in the blood, potentially reducing the risk of gout attacks. Drinking green tea regularly may be beneficial for individuals with gout, but more research is needed to confirm its efficacy.

10. Always Consult Your Healthcare Provider

Before using any herbal remedies for gout management, it's important to consult with your healthcare provider, especially if you have underlying health conditions or are taking medications. Your healthcare provider can help determine which herbal remedies may be appropriate for you and provide personalized recommendations based on your individual health needs and goals.

While herbal remedies may offer potential benefits for managing gout symptoms, they should not be used as a substitute for medical treatment or lifestyle changes recommended by your healthcare provider. Be sure to discuss any questions or concerns with your healthcare provider before using herbal remedies for gout management.

Consultation with Healthcare Providers for Gout Management

1. Comprehensive Assessment

Healthcare providers play a crucial role in the management of gout by conducting a comprehensive assessment of the patient's medical history, symptoms, lifestyle factors, and risk factors. This assessment helps healthcare providers develop an individualized treatment plan tailored to the patient's specific needs and goals.

2. Diagnosis Confirmation

Gout can mimic other conditions, and accurate diagnosis is essential for effective management. Healthcare providers use various diagnostic tools, such as blood tests, joint fluid analysis, and imaging studies, to confirm the diagnosis of gout and differentiate it from other forms of arthritis or inflammatory conditions.

3. Medication Management

Healthcare providers prescribe medications to manage gout symptoms, reduce inflammation, and lower uric acid levels in the blood. These medications may include nonsteroidal anti-inflammatory drugs (NSAIDs), colchicine, corticosteroids, and urate-lowering drugs (e.g., allopurinol, febuxostat). Healthcare providers monitor the patient's response to treatment and adjust medication regimens as needed to achieve optimal outcomes.

4. Lifestyle Counseling

Healthcare providers offer lifestyle counseling to individuals with gout to help them make positive changes in diet, exercise, and other lifestyle factors that can impact gout symptoms and disease progression. Lifestyle modifications, such as following a low-purine diet, maintaining a healthy weight, limiting alcohol consumption, and staying physically active, are key components of gout management.

5. Monitoring and Follow-Up

Healthcare providers monitor patients with gout regularly to assess treatment efficacy, evaluate disease progression, and address any new or worsening symptoms. Regular follow-up appointments allow healthcare providers to track changes in uric acid levels, assess medication tolerability, and provide ongoing support and guidance to patients.

6. Education and Empowerment

Healthcare providers educate patients about gout, its causes, symptoms, and treatment options, empowering them to take an active role in managing their condition. By providing accurate information and practical strategies for gout management, healthcare providers help patients make informed decisions about their health and well-being.

7. Preventive Care

Healthcare providers emphasize the importance of preventive care for individuals with gout to reduce the risk of gout attacks, complications, and comorbidities. This may include regular monitoring of uric acid levels, screening for associated conditions (e.g., hypertension, kidney disease), and implementing strategies to prevent future gout flares.

8. Coordination of Care

Healthcare providers collaborate with other members of the healthcare team, such as rheumatologists, primary care physicians, dietitians, and physical therapists, to ensure comprehensive and coordinated care for individuals with gout. This multidisciplinary approach helps address the diverse needs of patients and optimize treatment outcomes.

9. Patient-Centered Care

Healthcare providers prioritize patient-centered care, taking into account the individual preferences, values, and goals of each patient. By listening to patients' concerns, preferences, and treatment goals, healthcare providers can tailor treatment plans to meet their unique needs and preferences, fostering a collaborative and trusting relationship.

10. Importance of Communication

Effective communication between healthcare providers and patients is essential for successful gout management. Patients should feel comfortable discussing their symptoms, concerns, and treatment preferences with their healthcare providers, while healthcare providers should actively listen to patients' perspectives, address their questions and concerns, and provide clear and understandable information.

11. Always Consult Your Healthcare Provider

Individuals with gout should always consult their healthcare provider for personalized guidance, treatment recommendations, and ongoing support. Healthcare providers have the knowledge, expertise, and resources to help individuals with gout effectively manage their condition and improve their quality of life.

By seeking consultation with healthcare providers and actively participating in their care, individuals with gout can receive comprehensive, evidence-based treatment and support to effectively manage their condition and optimize their health outcomes.

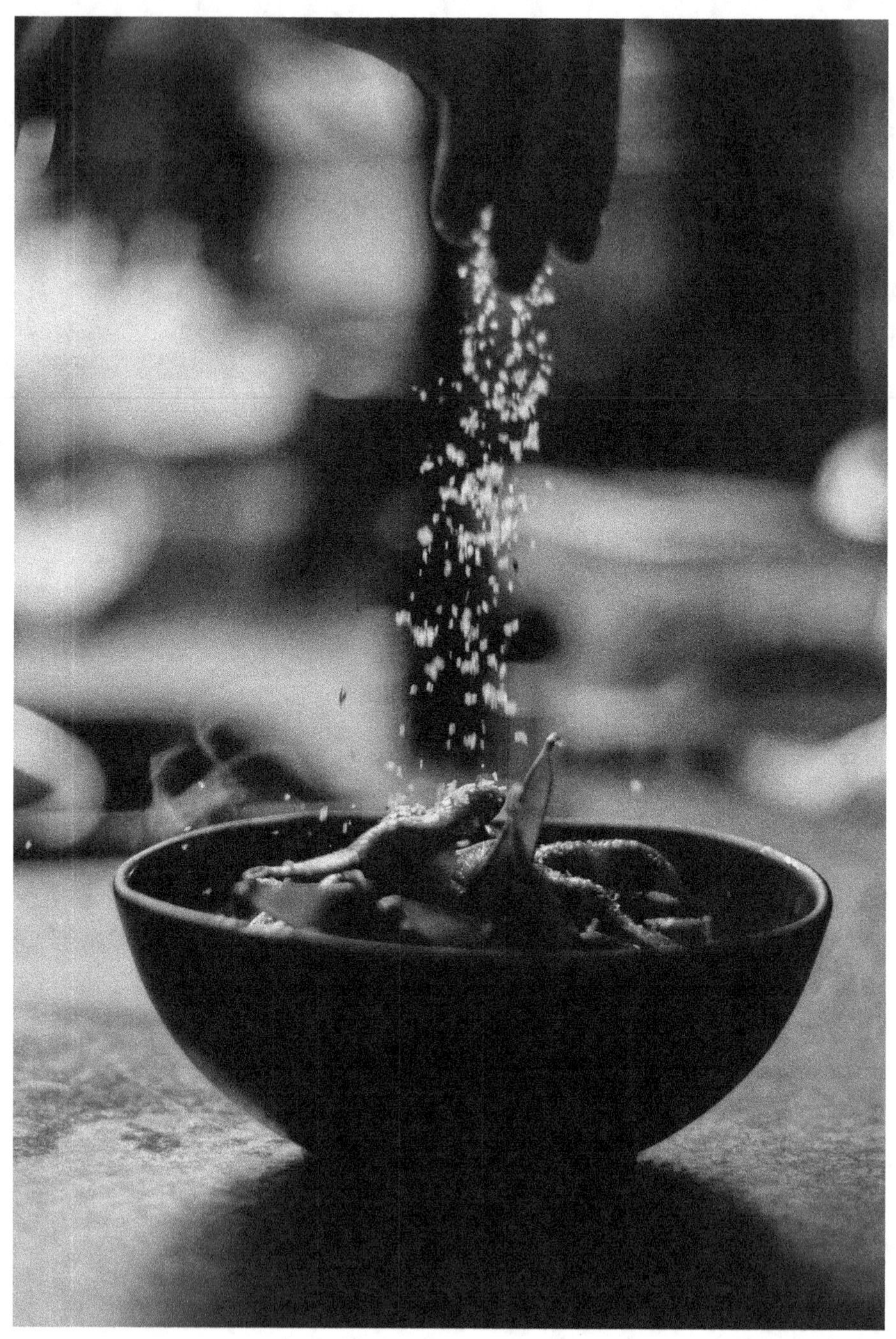

CHAPTER SIX

Coping with Gout Flares

Recognizing Gout Flares

Gout flares, also known as gout attacks or acute gouty arthritis, are sudden episodes of intense joint pain, swelling, redness, and tenderness caused by the deposition of urate crystals in the joints. Recognizing gout flares is essential for timely intervention and management. Here are some key signs and symptoms to watch for:

1. Sudden Onset of Joint Pain

Gout flares typically begin suddenly and without warning, often in the middle of the night or early morning. The pain is usually severe, intense, and localized to one joint, most commonly the big toe. However, gout can also affect other joints, such as the ankles, knees, elbows, wrists, and fingers.

2. Joint Swelling and Redness

Along with pain, gout flares often cause swelling, redness, warmth, and tenderness in the affected joint. The joint may appear visibly swollen and inflamed, and the skin over the joint may feel warm to the touch. The swelling and redness can make it difficult to move the joint and perform daily activities.

3. Limited Range of Motion

During a gout flare, the affected joint may become stiff and immobile, leading to a limited range of motion. Movements that involve the affected joint may be painful and may exacerbate symptoms. Individuals may experience difficulty walking, standing, or using the affected limb during a gout flare.

4. Increased Pain with Touch or Pressure

Gout flares can cause extreme sensitivity to touch or pressure in the affected joint. Even light pressure or contact with clothing or bedding may trigger intense pain and discomfort. Individuals may avoid touching or moving the affected joint due to the pain and tenderness.

5. Worsening Symptoms Over Hours to Days

Gout flares typically worsen over hours to days if left untreated, reaching peak intensity within 24-48 hours of onset. The pain and inflammation may gradually subside over the course of several days to weeks, but symptoms can persist for longer periods in some cases.

6. Associated Symptoms

In addition to joint symptoms, individuals experiencing a gout flare may also develop systemic symptoms such as fever, chills, fatigue, and malaise. These symptoms are more common in severe or prolonged flares and may indicate complications such as infection or systemic inflammation.

7. Triggers and Risk Factors

Gout flares can be triggered by various factors, including dietary indiscretions (e.g., consumption of high-purine foods, alcohol), dehydration, stress, trauma or injury to the joint, surgery, infection, and certain medications (e.g., diuretics, aspirin). Identifying and avoiding triggers can help reduce the frequency and severity of gout flares.

8. Differential Diagnosis

While gout flares have characteristic features, other conditions, such as infections, rheumatoid arthritis, pseudogout (calcium pyrophosphate deposition disease), and traumatic injury, can mimic gout and cause similar symptoms. It's important to consult a healthcare provider for accurate diagnosis and appropriate management.

9. Seek Medical Evaluation

If you experience symptoms suggestive of a gout flare, it's important to seek prompt medical evaluation from a healthcare provider. Your healthcare provider can perform a physical examination, order diagnostic tests (e.g., blood tests, joint aspiration), and provide appropriate treatment to alleviate symptoms and prevent future flares.

10. Long-Term Management

Managing gout involves both acute treatment of flares and long-term management to prevent future flares and complications. Lifestyle modifications, such as following a low-purine diet, maintaining a healthy weight, limiting alcohol consumption, and staying physically active, are essential for gout management. Medications may also be prescribed to lower uric acid levels and reduce the risk of flares.

Recognizing the signs and symptoms of gout flares is crucial for timely intervention and effective management. By staying vigilant and seeking prompt medical attention when symptoms occur, individuals with gout can better manage their condition and improve their quality of life.

Immediate Relief Measures for Gout Flares

1. Rest the Affected Joint

Resting the affected joint is crucial to reduce pain and inflammation during a gout flare. Avoid putting weight on the affected joint and elevate it whenever possible to help alleviate swelling and discomfort.

2. Apply Ice Packs

Applying ice packs to the affected joint can help reduce pain and inflammation during a gout flare. Wrap a cold pack or bag of ice in a thin towel and apply it to the affected joint for 15-20 minutes at a time, several times a day. Be sure to take breaks between icing sessions to prevent skin irritation.

3. Take Nonsteroidal Anti-Inflammatory Drugs (NSAIDs)

Over-the-counter NSAIDs, such as ibuprofen (Advil, Motrin) or naproxen (Aleve), can help reduce pain and inflammation associated with gout flares. Follow the recommended dosage instructions on the package, and consult your healthcare provider before taking NSAIDs if you have any underlying health conditions or are taking other medications.

4. Use Colchicine

Colchicine is a medication commonly used to treat acute gout flares. It works by reducing inflammation and pain associated with gout attacks. Your healthcare provider may prescribe colchicine to take at the first sign of a gout flare, typically in a higher dose followed by a lower maintenance dose.

5. Take Corticosteroids

Corticosteroids, such as prednisone or methylprednisolone, can be used to reduce inflammation and pain during severe gout flares. Corticosteroids may be taken orally, injected directly into the affected joint, or administered intravenously in a healthcare setting. Your healthcare provider will determine the appropriate dosage and route of administration based on your individual needs.

6. Stay Hydrated

Drinking plenty of water and staying hydrated can help flush excess uric acid from the body and alleviate gout symptoms. Aim to drink at least 8-10 glasses of water per day, and avoid sugary or caffeinated beverages, which can exacerbate dehydration.

7. Elevate the Affected Joint

Elevating the affected joint above the level of the heart can help reduce swelling and alleviate discomfort during a gout flare. Prop up the affected limb with pillows or cushions while resting to promote drainage of excess fluid from the joint.

8. Avoid Trigger Foods and Alcohol

During a gout flare, it's important to avoid trigger foods high in purines, such as red meat, organ meats, shellfish, and certain types of seafood (e.g., anchovies, sardines). Limiting alcohol consumption, particularly beer and spirits, can also help prevent exacerbation of gout symptoms.

9. Consider Herbal Remedies

Some herbal remedies, such as cherry extract, turmeric, and ginger, may have anti-inflammatory properties and could provide relief from gout symptoms. However, it's important to consult your healthcare provider before using herbal remedies, especially if you have any underlying health conditions or are taking other medications.

10. Follow Up with Healthcare Provider

If you experience a gout flare, it's important to follow up with your healthcare provider for further evaluation and management. Your healthcare provider can assess the severity of your symptoms, adjust your treatment plan as needed, and provide guidance on long-term management strategies to prevent future flares.

11. Monitor Symptoms

Pay attention to how your symptoms respond to treatment and monitor for any signs of complications, such as persistent swelling, fever, or difficulty moving the affected joint. If you experience worsening symptoms or new onset of symptoms, seek prompt medical attention.

12. Implement Long-Term Management Strategies

In addition to immediate relief measures, it's important to implement long-term management strategies to prevent future gout flares and complications. This may include lifestyle modifications, such as following a low-purine diet, maintaining a healthy weight, limiting alcohol consumption, and staying physically active, as well as taking medications to lower uric acid levels.

These immediate relief measures can help alleviate pain and inflammation during a gout flare. However, it's important to consult your healthcare provider for personalized guidance and treatment recommendations based on your individual needs and health status.

Long-Term Strategies for Managing Gout Flares

1. Follow a Low-Purine Diet

A low-purine diet can help reduce the production of uric acid in the body and minimize the risk of gout flares. Focus on consuming foods low in purines, such as fruits, vegetables, whole grains, and lean proteins. Limit intake of high-purine foods, including red meat, organ meats, shellfish, and certain types of seafood (e.g., anchovies, sardines).

2. Maintain a Healthy Weight

Maintaining a healthy weight is important for managing gout and reducing the frequency and severity of flares. Excess weight can increase uric acid levels in the blood and contribute to inflammation and joint damage. Aim to achieve and maintain a healthy weight through a combination of balanced diet, regular exercise, and lifestyle modifications.

3. Limit Alcohol Consumption

Alcohol, particularly beer and spirits, can exacerbate gout symptoms and increase the risk of flares. Limiting alcohol consumption or avoiding alcohol altogether can help prevent gout flares and improve overall gout management. If you choose to drink alcohol, do so in moderation and consider opting for lower-purine options, such as clear spirits like vodka or gin.

4. Stay Hydrated

Drinking plenty of water and staying hydrated can help flush excess uric acid from the body and reduce the risk of gout flares. Aim to drink at least 8-10 glasses of water per day, and avoid sugary or caffeinated beverages, which can exacerbate dehydration. Be mindful of your fluid intake, especially during hot weather or when engaging in physical activity.

5. Take Medications as Prescribed

Medications are often prescribed to manage gout symptoms and prevent future flares. Urate-lowering drugs, such as allopurinol or febuxostat, help reduce uric acid levels in the blood and lower the risk of gout flares over time. Take your medications as prescribed by your healthcare provider, and follow up regularly to monitor your response to treatment and adjust your medication regimen as needed.

6. Manage Comorbidities

Certain comorbidities, such as hypertension, diabetes, and kidney disease, can exacerbate gout and increase the risk of flares. Managing underlying health conditions through lifestyle modifications, medications, and regular medical care can help improve gout management and reduce the frequency of flares.

7. Avoid Trigger Factors

Identify and avoid trigger factors that may contribute to gout flares, such as dietary indiscretions, dehydration, stress, trauma or injury to the joint, surgery, infection, and certain medications (e.g., diuretics, aspirin). Making lifestyle modifications and avoiding triggers can help minimize the risk of gout flares and improve overall gout management.

8. Monitor Uric Acid Levels

Regular monitoring of uric acid levels in the blood can help assess the effectiveness of treatment and identify individuals at risk of gout flares. Your healthcare provider may recommend periodic blood tests to measure uric acid levels and adjust your treatment plan accordingly to maintain optimal uric acid control.

9. Incorporate Regular Physical Activity

Regular physical activity can help improve gout management by promoting weight loss, reducing inflammation, and enhancing overall health and well-being. Aim for at least 150 minutes of moderate-intensity aerobic activity or 75 minutes of vigorous-intensity aerobic activity per week, along with muscle-strengthening exercises on two or more days per week.

10. Educate Yourself About Gout

Educating yourself about gout, its causes, symptoms, triggers, and treatment options can empower you to make informed decisions about your health and well-being. Work closely with your healthcare provider to develop a personalized management plan tailored to your individual needs and goals.

11. Practice Stress Management

Stress can exacerbate inflammation and trigger gout flares in some individuals. Practice stress management techniques, such as deep breathing exercises, meditation, yoga, tai chi, or mindfulness, to reduce stress and promote relaxation. Incorporating stress management techniques into your daily routine can help improve gout management and reduce the risk of flares.

12. Seek Support and Guidance

Managing gout can be challenging, but you don't have to do it alone. Seek support and guidance from your healthcare provider, rheumatologist, dietitian, physical therapist, or support groups for individuals with gout. Surround yourself with a supportive network of healthcare professionals and peers who can provide encouragement, guidance, and practical strategies for managing gout effectively.

By implementing these long-term strategies for managing gout flares, you can reduce the frequency and severity of flares, improve overall gout management, and enhance your quality of life.

Common Questions About Gout

1. What is gout?

Gout is a type of inflammatory arthritis caused by the deposition of urate crystals in the joints, leading to sudden and severe episodes of joint pain, swelling, redness, and tenderness. Gout most commonly affects the big toe, but it can also affect other joints, such as the ankles, knees, elbows, wrists, and fingers.

2. What causes gout?

Gout is caused by elevated levels of uric acid in the blood, a condition known as hyperuricemia. Uric acid is a waste product that forms when the body breaks down purines, which are found in certain foods and beverages. When uric acid levels are high, urate crystals can form and accumulate in the joints, triggering gout flares.

3. What are the risk factors for gout?

Several factors can increase the risk of developing gout, including:

Genetics: Family history of gout or inherited disorders affecting uric acid metabolism.

Diet: Consumption of purine-rich foods (e.g., red meat, organ meats, shellfish), sugary beverages, and alcohol, particularly beer and spirits.

Obesity: Excess body weight can lead to higher uric acid levels and increase the risk of gout.

Medical Conditions: Conditions such as hypertension, diabetes, kidney disease, and metabolic syndrome can increase the risk of gout.

Medications: Certain medications, such as diuretics, aspirin, and immunosuppressants, can raise uric acid levels and trigger gout flares.

4. How is gout diagnosed?

Gout is diagnosed based on a combination of clinical symptoms, medical history, physical examination, and diagnostic tests. Healthcare providers may perform blood tests to measure uric acid levels, joint fluid analysis to detect urate crystals in the affected joint, and imaging studies (e.g., X-rays, ultrasound) to assess joint damage and rule out other conditions.

5. What are the symptoms of a gout flare?

Symptoms of a gout flare include sudden and intense joint pain, swelling, redness, warmth, and tenderness in the affected joint. The pain is often described as throbbing, excruciating, and debilitating, and can make it difficult to walk, stand, or use the affected limb. Gout flares typically occur suddenly, often at night or in the early morning, and can last for several days to weeks if left untreated.

6. How are gout flares treated?

Gout flares are typically treated with medications to relieve pain and inflammation, such as nonsteroidal anti-inflammatory drugs (NSAIDs), colchicine, and corticosteroids. Rest, ice packs, elevation of the affected joint, and staying hydrated can also help alleviate symptoms during a gout flare. In some cases, healthcare providers may recommend urate-lowering drugs to prevent future flares.

7. Can gout be cured?

Gout is a chronic condition that requires ongoing management to prevent flares and complications. While there is no cure for gout, lifestyle modifications, medications, and dietary changes can help control symptoms, reduce the frequency of flares, and improve quality of life. With proper treatment and management, many individuals with gout can lead active and fulfilling lives.

8. How can gout be prevented?

To prevent gout flares and manage the condition effectively, individuals can take the following steps:

Follow a balanced diet low in purines and rich in fruits, vegetables, whole grains, and lean proteins.

Maintain a healthy weight through diet and regular exercise.

Limit alcohol consumption, particularly beer and spirits.

Stay hydrated by drinking plenty of water throughout the day.

Avoid trigger factors that may exacerbate gout symptoms, such as certain foods, beverages, medications, and stress.

Take medications as prescribed by your healthcare provider to lower uric acid levels and prevent future flares.

9. When should I see a healthcare provider for gout?

It's important to seek medical attention if you experience symptoms suggestive of gout, such as sudden and severe joint pain, swelling, redness, and tenderness. Your healthcare provider can perform a thorough evaluation, diagnose the underlying cause of your symptoms, and recommend appropriate treatment to alleviate pain and prevent future flares. Additionally, if you have been diagnosed with gout and experience worsening symptoms, new onset of symptoms, or complications, it's essential to follow up with your healthcare provider for further evaluation and management.

10. Can gout affect other parts of the body besides the joints?

While gout primarily affects the joints, it can also lead to complications affecting other parts of the body, such as the kidneys, skin, and soft tissues. Chronic hyperuricemia can contribute to the formation of urate crystals in the kidneys, leading to kidney stones or gouty nephropathy (kidney damage). In some cases, urate crystals can deposit in the skin, causing nodules called tophi. Rarely, gout can affect other organs, such as the heart and lungs, leading to serious complications.

These are just a few common questions about gout and their answers. If you have additional questions or concerns about gout, it's important to consult your healthcare provider for personalized guidance and support.

Addressing Misconceptions About Gout

Misconception 1: Gout only affects elderly men.
Clarification: While gout is more common in older adults and men, it can affect individuals of any age, gender, or demographic group. Women, younger adults, and even children can develop gout, although it is less common in these populations.

Misconception 2: Gout is solely caused by diet.
Clarification: While diet plays a role in gout development and management, it is not the sole cause of the condition. Gout is primarily caused by elevated levels of uric acid in the blood, which can result from a combination of genetic factors, lifestyle habits, medical conditions, and medication use.

Misconception 3: All high-protein foods should be avoided in gout.
Clarification: While some high-protein foods, such as red meat and organ meats, are rich in purines and may contribute to gout flares in susceptible individuals, not all high-protein foods are off-limits. Lean proteins, such as poultry, fish, tofu, and legumes, can be included in a gout-friendly diet in moderation.

Misconception 4: Gout is just a temporary inconvenience.
Clarification: Gout is a chronic condition that requires ongoing management to prevent flares and complications. Without proper

treatment and lifestyle modifications, gout can lead to recurrent flares, joint damage, and other health problems over time.

Misconception 5: Only medications can lower uric acid levels.
Clarification: While medications such as allopurinol, febuxostat, and probenecid are commonly used to lower uric acid levels in the blood, lifestyle modifications can also play a significant role in managing gout. Following a low-purine diet, maintaining a healthy weight, limiting alcohol consumption, staying hydrated, and exercising regularly can help lower uric acid levels and reduce the risk of gout flares.

Misconception 6: Gout is just a joint problem.
Clarification: While gout primarily affects the joints, it can also lead to complications affecting other parts of the body, such as the kidneys, skin, and soft tissues. Chronic hyperuricemia can contribute to the formation of kidney stones, gouty nephropathy (kidney damage), and skin nodules called tophi. Gout can also increase the risk of cardiovascular disease and other systemic conditions.

Misconception 7: Once you start urate-lowering medication, you no longer need to make lifestyle changes.
Clarification: Urate-lowering medications, such as allopurinol or febuxostat, are effective for lowering uric acid levels and reducing the frequency of gout flares. However, lifestyle modifications remain an important component of gout management, even when taking medication. Following a healthy diet, maintaining a healthy weight, limiting alcohol consumption, staying hydrated, and exercising regularly can complement medication therapy and improve overall gout control.

Misconception 8: Gout is a sign of excessive drinking.

Clarification: While excessive alcohol consumption, particularly of beer and spirits, can increase the risk of gout flares in some individuals, not all people with gout are heavy drinkers. Gout can occur in individuals with moderate or even minimal alcohol intake, and there are many other factors that contribute to its development, including genetics, diet, obesity, medical conditions, and medication use.

Misconception 9: Gout is just a minor inconvenience and doesn't require medical attention.

Clarification: Gout can cause significant pain, disability, and impairment of quality of life if left untreated or poorly managed. Recurrent gout flares can lead to joint damage, deformity, and functional limitations. Seeking medical attention and following a comprehensive treatment plan are essential for effectively managing gout and preventing long-term complications.

Misconception 10: Natural remedies can cure gout.

Clarification: While certain natural remedies, such as cherry extract, turmeric, and ginger, may have anti-inflammatory properties and could provide relief from gout symptoms, they are not a cure for gout. Gout is a chronic condition that requires ongoing management, including medication therapy, lifestyle modifications, and regular medical care, to control symptoms and prevent flares.

Addressing these misconceptions about gout can help promote accurate understanding and facilitate effective management of the condition.

Real-Life Success Stories of Gout Management

1. John's Journey to Better Health

John, a 52-year-old man, struggled with recurrent gout flares for years, which severely impacted his ability to work and enjoy life. Determined to take control of his health, John sought guidance from a rheumatologist and a registered dietitian. With their support, he made significant lifestyle changes, including adopting a low-purine diet, losing weight through regular exercise, and limiting alcohol consumption. John also started taking urate-lowering medication to lower his uric acid levels. Over time, John experienced fewer gout flares, improved mobility, and increased energy levels. Today, he enjoys an active lifestyle, free from the debilitating pain of gout.

2. Sarah's Struggle and Triumph

Sarah, a 38-year-old woman, was diagnosed with gout after experiencing severe joint pain and swelling in her feet and ankles. As a busy working mother, Sarah found it challenging to manage her gout while juggling family and career responsibilities. With the help of her healthcare provider and a supportive network of family and friends, Sarah embarked on a journey to better health. She made gradual changes to her diet, focusing on incorporating more fruits, vegetables, whole grains, and lean proteins while avoiding trigger foods high in purines. Sarah also prioritized regular exercise, stress management techniques, and staying hydrated. Through perseverance and dedication, Sarah was able to significantly reduce the frequency and severity of her gout flares, allowing her to live a more fulfilling and active life.

3. Mark's Transformation Through Education

Mark, a 45-year-old man, struggled with gout for years without fully understanding the underlying causes and triggers of his condition. After attending a gout education seminar led by a team of healthcare professionals, Mark gained valuable insights into the importance of diet, lifestyle, and medication management in controlling gout. Armed with this knowledge, Mark made informed decisions about his health and implemented practical strategies to manage his gout effectively. He learned to identify and avoid trigger foods, stay hydrated, maintain a healthy weight, and take his medication as prescribed. As a result, Mark experienced fewer gout flares, improved mobility, and enhanced overall well-being. Inspired by his success, Mark became an advocate for gout awareness, sharing his story and empowering others to take charge of their health.

4. Maria's Journey to Optimal Health

Maria, a 60-year-old woman, struggled with gout and its associated complications for many years, including kidney stones and tophi. Frustrated by the limitations imposed by her condition, Maria sought comprehensive care from a multidisciplinary team of healthcare providers, including rheumatologists, nephrologists, and dietitians. Together, they developed a personalized treatment plan tailored to Maria's unique needs and goals. Maria made significant lifestyle changes, including following a strict low-purine diet, staying hydrated, and adhering to her medication regimen. With ongoing support and encouragement from her healthcare team, Maria achieved optimal control of her gout, experienced fewer flares, and improved her kidney function. Today, Maria enjoys an active and fulfilling life, free from the burden of gout and its complications.

These real-life success stories illustrate the transformative power of education, support, and personalized care in managing gout effectively and improving quality of life.

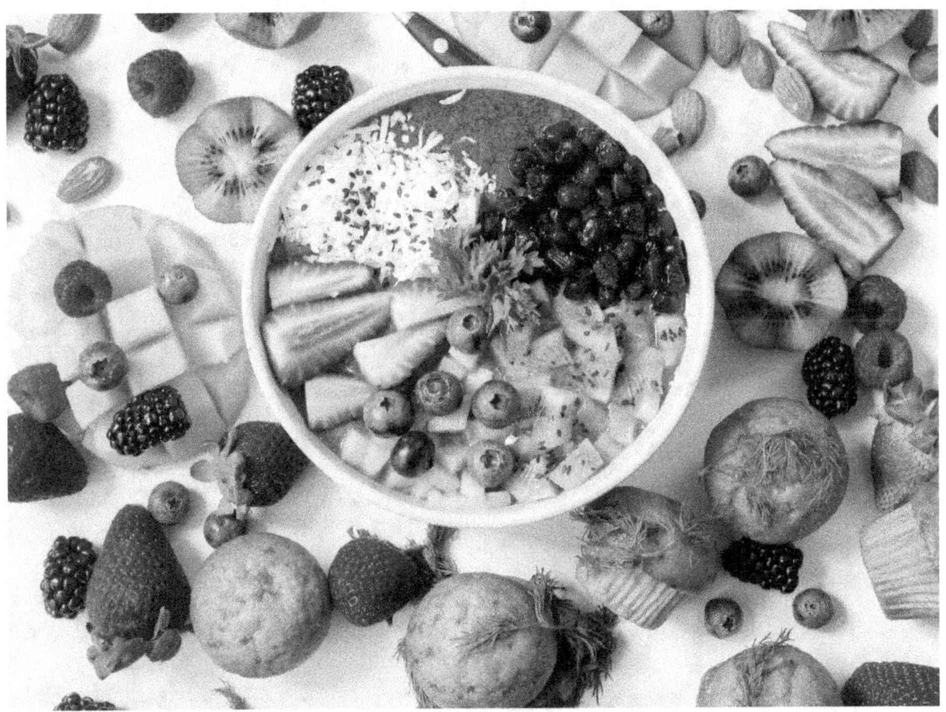

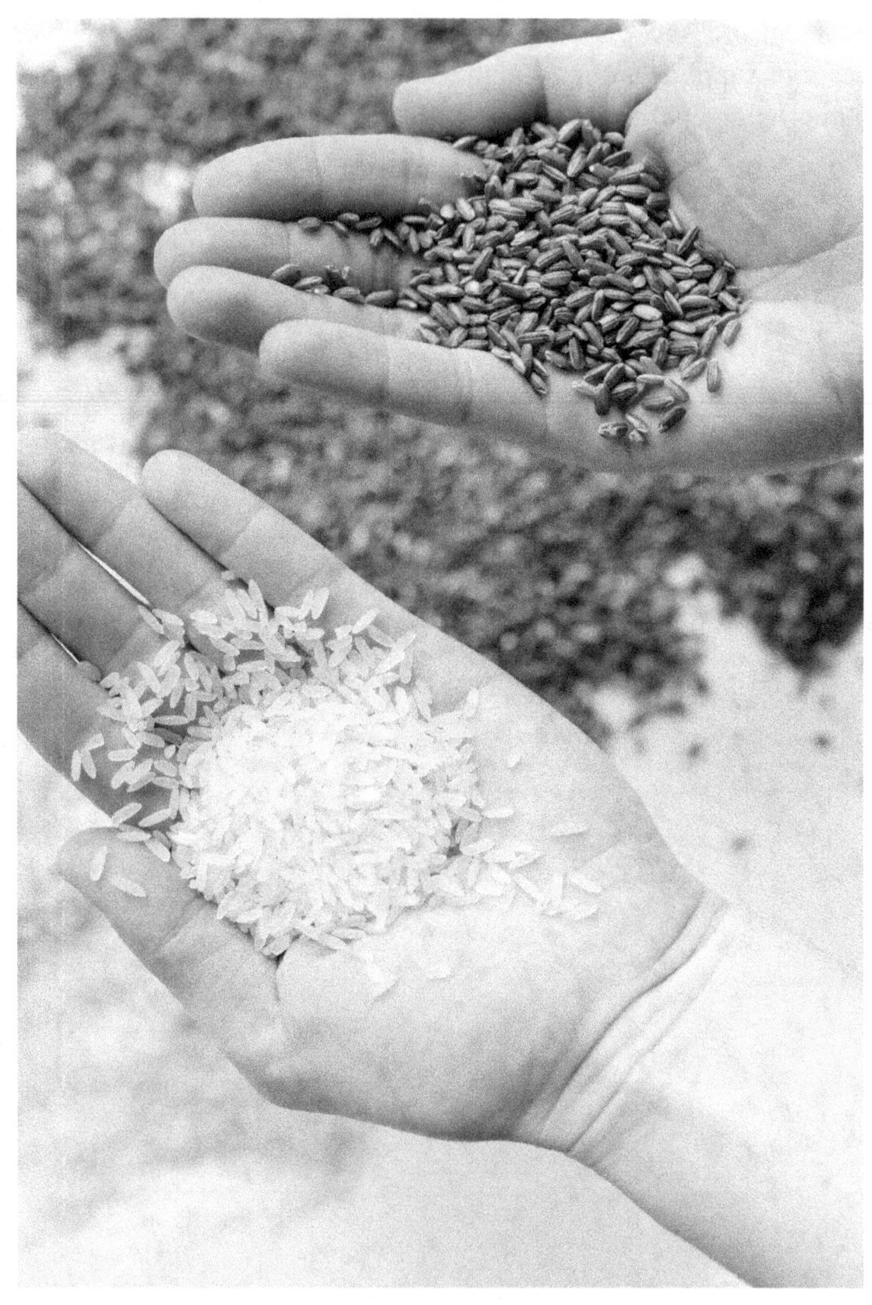

CONCLUSION

FAQs and Common Concerns

Final Thoughts

Living with gout can be challenging, but with proper education, support, and management strategies, individuals can effectively control their symptoms and improve their quality of life. Gout is a chronic condition characterized by recurrent flares of joint pain, swelling, and inflammation, caused by the deposition of urate crystals in the joints. While gout primarily affects the joints, it can also lead to complications affecting other parts of the body, such as the kidneys, skin, and soft tissues.

Managing gout requires a comprehensive approach that addresses both acute flares and long-term prevention. Lifestyle modifications, such as following a low-purine diet, maintaining a healthy weight, limiting alcohol consumption, staying hydrated, and exercising regularly, play a crucial role in gout management. Medications, such as NSAIDs, colchicine, corticosteroids, and urate-lowering drugs, may also be prescribed to alleviate symptoms and prevent future flares.

In addition to medical interventions, education and support are essential components of successful gout management. By understanding the underlying causes of gout, identifying trigger factors, and learning effective self-care strategies, individuals can take an active role in managing their condition and reducing the risk of flares and complications. Seeking guidance from healthcare providers, participating in gout education programs, and connecting with peer support groups can provide valuable resources and encouragement along the journey.

It's important to remember that managing gout is not a one-size-fits-all approach. Each individual may respond differently to treatment, and what works for one person may not work for another. It may take time and patience to find the right combination of lifestyle modifications and medications that work best for you. By working closely with your healthcare provider and staying committed to your treatment plan, you can achieve optimal control of your gout and enjoy a better quality of life.

In closing, gout is a manageable condition that requires proactive management and ongoing commitment to healthy living. By taking control of your health, seeking support from healthcare professionals and peers, and staying informed about your condition, you can overcome the challenges of gout and live life to the fullest.

If you have any further questions or need additional assistance, feel free to reach out. Wishing you all the best on your journey to managing gout effectively!

Resources for Further Reading

1. Arthritis Foundation: Gout
Website: Arthritis Foundation
The Arthritis Foundation provides comprehensive information on gout, including symptoms, causes, risk factors, diagnosis, treatment options, and lifestyle recommendations. The website also offers educational

resources, support programs, and advocacy initiatives for individuals living with gout.

2. Centers for Disease Control and Prevention (CDC): Gout
Website: CDC - Gout

The CDC offers evidence-based information on gout, including prevalence, risk factors, complications, and public health initiatives aimed at preventing and managing the condition. The website also provides resources for healthcare professionals, policymakers, and the general public.

3. American College of Rheumatology (ACR): Gout
Website: ACR - Gout

The American College of Rheumatology offers patient-friendly resources on gout, including educational articles, treatment guidelines, and tips for managing symptoms. The website also provides information on finding a rheumatologist and accessing rheumatology care.

4. Mayo Clinic: Gout
Website: Mayo Clinic - Gout

Mayo Clinic offers reliable information on gout, including symptoms, causes, diagnosis, treatment options, and lifestyle recommendations. The website also features patient stories, expert Q&A sessions, and interactive tools for assessing gout risk and tracking symptoms.

5. National Institute of Arthritis and Musculoskeletal and Skin Diseases (NIAMS): Gout
Website: NIAMS - Gout

NIAMS provides in-depth resources on gout, including research updates, clinical trials, and patient education materials. The website also offers information on related conditions, such as hyperuricemia, and links to additional resources from the National Institutes of Health (NIH).

6. Gout & Uric Acid Education Society
Website: Gout & Uric Acid Education Society
The Gout & Uric Acid Education Society is dedicated to raising awareness about gout and hyperuricemia through education, advocacy, and research. The website features educational videos, patient testimonials, and downloadable resources for healthcare providers and patients.

www.ingramcontent.com/pod-product-compliance
Lightning Source LLC
Chambersburg PA
CBHW070810260726
48660CB00005B/1797